Current Concepts of Treatment of Metatarsalgia

Editor

GASTÓN SLULLITEL

FOOT AND ANKLE CLINICS

www.foot.theclinics.com

Consulting Editor
MARK S. MYERSON

December 2019 • Volume 24 • Number 4

ELSEVIER

1600 John F. Kennedy Boulevard • Suite 1800 • Philadelphia, Pennsylvania, 19103-2899

http://www.theclinics.com

FOOT AND ANKLE CLINICS Volume 24, Number 4
December 2019 ISSN 1083-7515, ISBN-978-0-323-72210-0

Editor: Lauren Boyle
Developmental Editor: Donald Mumford

Foot and Ankle Clinics (ISSN 1083-7515) is published quarterly by Elsevier, Inc., 360 Park Avenue South, New York, NY 10010-1710. Months of issue are March, June, September, and December. Periodicals postage paid at New York, NY, and additional mailing offices. Subscription price per year is $337.00 (US individuals), $552.00 (US institutions), $100.00 (US students), $371.00 (Canadian individuals), $663.00 (Canadian institutions), $215.00 (Canadian students), $465.00 (international individuals), $663.00 (international institutions), and $215.00 (international students). To receive student/resident rate, orders must be accompanied by name of affiliated institution, date of term, and the *signature* of program/residency coordinator on institution letterhead. Orders will be billed at individual rate until proof of status is received. Foreign air speed delivery is included in all *Clinics* subscription prices. All prices are subject to change without notice. **POSTMASTER:** Send address changes to *Foot and Ankle Clinics*, Elsevier Health Sciences Division, Subscription Customer Service, 3251 Riverport Lane, Maryland Heights, MO 63043. **Customer Service: 1-800-654-2452 (US and Canada). From outside of the United States and Canada, call 314-447-8871. Fax: 314-447-8029. E-mail: JournalsCustomerService-usa@ elsevier.com (for print support); JournalsOnlineSupport-usa@elsevier.com (for online support).**

Reprints. For copies of 100 or more, of articles in this publication, please contact the Commercial Reprints Department, Elsevier Inc., 360 Park Avenue South, New York, NY 10010-1710. Tel.: 212-633-3874; Fax: 212-633-3820; E-mail: reprints@elsevier.com.

Contributors

CONSULTING EDITOR

MARK S. MYERSON, MD
Executive Director, Steps2Walk, Miami, Florida, USA

EDITOR

GASTÓN SLULLITEL, MD
Chief, Department of Foot and Ankle Surgery, J Slullitel Institute of Orthopedics, Rosario, Santa Fe, Argentina

AUTHORS

AMIETHAB AIYER, MD
Chief of Foot & Ankle Service, University of Miami Miller School of Medicine, Miami, Florida, USA

JUAN PABLO CALVI, MD
Department of Foot and Ankle Surgery, J Slullitel Institute of Orthopedics, Rosario, Santa Fe, Argentina

NORMAN ESPINOSA, MD
Institute for Foot and Ankle Reconstruction, FussInsitut Zurich, Zurich, Switzerland

RODRIGO MOTA PACHECO FERNANDES, MD
CALO -Centro de Alongamento Ósseo, Rio de Janeiro, Brazil

JAVIER Z. GUZMAN, MD
House Staff, The Mount Sinai Hospital, Mount Sinai West, Leni & Peter W. May Department of Orthopedic Surgery, Icahn School of Medicine at Mount Sinai, New York, New York, USA

THOMAS G. HARRIS, MD
Congress Orthopedic Associates, Pasadena, California, USA; Chief, Foot and Ankle Surgery, UCLA Harbor Medical Center, Torrance, California, USA

GEORG KLAMMER, MD
Institute for Foot and Ankle Reconstruction, Zurich, Switzerland

OLIVIER LAFFENÊTRE, MD
Foot & Ankle Institute, Paris, France; Lecturer, Bordeaux 2 University, Founding Member of GRECMIP, University Medico-Surgical Foot Center, Pellegrin University Hospital, Bordeaux, France

JAVIER SERRANO LARA, MD
Trauma and Orthopaedic Department, Hospital de Rengo, Rengo, Chile

VALERIA LOPEZ, MD
Deparment of Foot and Ankle Surgery, J Slullitel Institute of Orthopaedics, Rosario, Santa Fe, Argentina

ERNESTO MACEIRA, MD
Orthopaedic Foot and Ankle Unit, Complejo Hospitalario La Mancha Centro, Alcázar de San Juan, Ciudad Real, Spain

MANUEL MONTEAGUDO, MD
Orthopaedic Foot and Ankle Unit, Orthopaedic and Trauma Department, Hospital Universitario Quirónsalud Madrid, Faculty Medicine UEM Madrid, Madrid, Spain

ANTHONY PERERA, MBChB, FRCS(Orth)
Consultant Orthopaedic Foot and Ankle Surgeon, Spire Cardiff Hospital, Cardiff, Wales, United Kingdom

SUDHEER C. REDDY, MD
Department of Orthopaedic Surgery, Shady Grove Orthopaedics, Adventist Health Care, George Washington School of Medicine, Rockville, Maryland, USA

ANDRÉ PERIN SHECAIRA, MD
Foot and Ankle Medical Staff, Instituto Nacional de Traumatologia e Ortopedia, Rio de Janeiro, Brazil

GASTÓN SLULLITEL, MD
Chief, Department of Foot and Ankle Surgery, J Slullitel Institute of Orthopedics, Rosario, Santa Fe, Argentina

HANS-JÖRG TRNKA, MD
Director, Foot and Ankle Center, Vienna, Austria; Professor, University of Vienna Medical School, Vienna, Austria

MATTHEW VARACALLO, MD
Chief of Sports Medicine Service, Department of Orthopaedic Surgery and Sports Medicine, Penn Highlands Healthcare System, DuBois, Pennsylvania, USA

ETTORE VULCANO, MD
Assistant Professor of Orthopaedics, Chief of Orthopedic Foot and Ankle Surgery, Mount Sinai West, Leni & Peter W. May Department of Orthopedic Surgery, Icahn School of Medicine at Mount Sinai, New York, New York, USA

ANGELA K. WALKER, DO
Orthopedic Surgeons, Inc, Kansas City, Missouri, USA

Editorial Advisory Board

Contents

Historically, metatarsalgia was approached as a forefoot condition, most often associated with hallux valgus. Consequently, surgical treatments were limited to that anatomic zone, disregarding more proximal structures. In order to assess this entity properly, it is necessary to consider anatomic and biomechanical factors, as well as general and local conditions of the affected patients. A thorough understanding of the multiple potential causal factors is essential to ensure selection of the optimal treatment.

 Video content accompanies this article at http://www.foot.theclinics.com.

The 3-rocker mechanism of gait provides a framework to understand why patients have mechanical metatarsal pain and to differentiate between the various types of metatarsalgia. Clinical examination of the patient together with radiological findings allows identification of the type of metatarsalgia and the pathomechanics involved, and the planning of surgical treatment. Second-rocker/nonpropulsive metatarsalgia is related with an abnormal inclination of a metatarsal in the sagittal plane, either anatomic or functional (equinism). Third-rocker/propulsive metatarsalgia is related to an abnormal length of a certain metatarsal with respect to the neighboring metatarsals in the transverse plane.

Metatarsalgia is a common foot disease with a multitude of causes. Proper identification of underlying diseases is mandatory to formulate an adequate treatment. Multiple surgical solutions are available to treat metatarsalgia. Only limited scientific evidence is available in the literature. However, most of the techniques used in the treatment of metatarsalgia seem to be reasonable with acceptable results.

Weil osteotomy (WO) is the most common technique worldwide for the treatment of mechanical metatarsalgia. The main indication for WO is propulsive/third rocker metatarsalgia that is in relation with an abnormal length of a certain metatarsal with respect to the neighboring metatarsals in the frontal plane. Most clinical studies have showed good to excellent results after WO. However, complications such as floating toes led to evolution of WO and the development of the triple-cut WO that allows for shortening coaxial to the shaft without plantar translation of metatarsal head. Other variations of WO may treat other forefoot disorders.

The use of a Shannon burr facilitates an osteotomy of the lesser metatarsals without requiring an open approach to the metatarsal. The end result that is aimed for is the same as for open surgery and therefore care needs to be taken to perform the bone cut in the appropriate manner. A description is provided of the surgical technique for distal minimally invasive osteotomy and its newer modifications—the distal intracapsular minimally invasive osteotomy and the distal oblique metatarsal osteotomy.

Advancements in lesser metatarsophalangeal (MTP) instability have involved the use of minimally invasive surgery techniques, synthetic augmentation of existing transfers, and use of arthroscopy for both diagnosing and addressing MTP disorder. Advances in imaging modalities, particularly MRI, have aided in diagnosing subtle instability. Clinical outcomes seem to be similar to traditional approaches as the indications and applicability continue to evolve.

Two theories exist in the development of central or transfer metatarsalgia. First, as the severity of hallux valgus increases, there is mechanical overload of the second metatarsal. Second, increased relative lesser metatarsal length is thought to contribute to metatarsalgia. It is imperative, in the treatment of first ray disorders (hallux valgus or hallux rigidus), to not overshorten the first ray when addressing the first ray pathologic condition. Treatment of metatarsalgia in the setting of failed hallux valgus correction can be treated with both conservative and surgical options.

A fundamental etiologic component of metatarsalgia is the repetitive loading of a locally concentrated force in the forefoot during gait. In the setting of an isolated gastrocnemius contracture, weight-bearing pressure is shifted toward the forefoot. If metatarsalgia is considered an entity more than a symptom, evaluation of gastrocnemius contracture must be a part of the physical examination, and gastrocnemius recession via the Baumann procedure alone, or in combination with other procedures, considered as an alternative treatment in an attempt to restore normal foot biomechanics.

Metatarsus adductus (MA) is a congenital condition resulting in adduction of the forefoot at the tarsometatarsal joint, medial metatarsal deviation, supination of the hindfoot through the subtalar joint, and plantarflexed first ray. The exact underlying pathophysiology remains elusive. There is increasing evidence highlighting the importance of recognizing MA as an associated deformity that complicates management of hallux valgus (HV). Unfortunately, metatarsalgia and lesser toe pathology is also common in this population. We present a review regarding the epidemiology, pathomechanics, and a comprehensive surgical treatment algorithm to optimize the management of patients with MA, HV, lesser toe deformity, and metatarsalgia.

Freiberg's infraction is an uncommon condition of the lesser metatarsophalangeal joints. Onset is usually between the 11th and 17th year of age. It is the only osteochondrosis that dominantly affects females with a reported female-to-male ratio of 5.1. The second metatarsal is most frequently involved (68%) followed by the third metatarsal (27%), and the fourth (3%). Surgical treatment options can be categorized in joint destructive and joint preserving procedures. Studies reveal complete resolution of pain and full return to activities in 70% after joint destructive procedure and more than 90% after joint preserving procedures.

Brachymetatarsia is a rare deformity with controversial clinical presentation. Multiple acute and gradual lengthening surgical techniques have been described for correction of this type of foot deformity. All techniques try to create a better appearance, facilitate shoeing, or solve possible transfer metatarsalgia. Either acute lengthening (1-stage procedure) or gradual lengthening (2 stages) is selected based on the patient's deformities, concerns, and clinical needs.

Resection arthroplasty for metatarsalgia is a selective procedure primarily indicated for patients with rheumatoid arthritis. These patients present with significant forefoot deformities, poor bone quality, and loss of soft tissue integrity. Resection of the metatarsal heads and correction of lesser toe deformities improve pain and decrease transfer metatarsalgia. Patients with concurrent hallux valgus may benefit from a lapidus procedure or hallux metatarsophalangeal fusion in an effort to improve outcomes and decrease incidence of recurrent hallux valgus. In rare cases, diabetics with neuropathy may require resection arthroplasty in the setting of forefoot deformities recalcitrant to other modalities.

FOOT AND ANKLE CLINICS

RELATED SERIES

Clinics in Sports Medicine
Orthopedic Clinics
Physical Medicine and Rehabilitation Clinics

THE CLINICS ARE NOW AVAILABLE ONLINE!
Access your subscription at:
www.theclinics.com

FOOT AND ANKLE CLINICS

FORTHCOMING ISSUES

March 2020
Current Controversies in the Approach to
Complex Hallux Valgus Deformity
Correction
Andrew Belis, Editor

June 2020
Correction of Lesser Toe and Soft Tissue
Deformities
Andy Molloy, Editor

September 2020
Advances in Minimally Invasive Surgery
Anthony Perera, Editor

RECENT ISSUES

September 2019
Updates in the Management of Acute and
Chronic Lesions of the Achilles Tendon
Phinit Phisitkul, Editor

June 2019
The Cavus Foot

March 2019
Avascular Necrosis of the Foot and Ankle
Kenneth J. Hunt, Editor

RELATED SERIES

Foot & Ankle Clinics
Orthopedic Clinics
Physical Medicine and Rehabilitation Clinics

Preface

Current Concepts of Treatment of Metatarsalgia

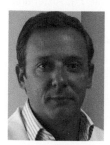

Gastón Slullitel, MD
Editor

Metatarsalgia is a frequent complaint in our day-to-day practice. Unfortunately, sometimes we face the frustrating scenario of dealing with an unpredictable malady. This situation is probably explained by the fact that constitutes a complex entity that is not enough appraised.

In our training stage, we all learned the diagnostic and therapeutic tools to manage this disorder. This includes the classical concepts that constitute the rationale of this pathologic condition. However, there is little high-level evidence (level I) to support the majority of the procedures that are commonly performed.

Consequently, expert opinion appears to be a very valuable source of knowledge, and *Foot and Ankle Clinics* brings a unique opportunity to provide an interesting support for foot and ankle surgeons. These include secrets, tricks, and subtle aspects about this topic.

Since many diagnostic and therapeutic aspects remain unknown, it is a great occasion to bring new ideas that will help to improve our patients. Forefoot surgery is full of controversial topics (eg, open vs minimally invasive surgery), and therefore, I would like to promote a pragmatic and unbiased view of metatarsalgia in order to develop new treatment strategies.

I thank all my colleagues participating in this project, for providing excellent insight and updating important aspects of metatarsalgia. A very special thanks goes to Mark Myerson, my friend and teacher, for his kind invitation to serve as guest editor of this issue. He generously shared with me his knowledge and taught me how to "read between the lines."

I am also grateful to Atilio Migues and Luis Muscolo, my mentors, who profoundly influenced in my career. Finally, I also thank Meredith Madeira and all the Elsevier staff for helping me during the publication process.

Foot Ankle Clin N Am 24 (2019) xiii–xiv
https://doi.org/10.1016/j.fcl.2019.09.001
1083-7515/19/© 2019 Published by Elsevier Inc.

foot.theclinics.com

I hope this issue will help foot and ankle surgeons to comprehensively approach metatarsalgia and stimulate the discovery of new ideas in order to improve the care of our patients.

Gastón Slullitel, MD
Department of Foot and Ankle Surgery
J Slullitel Institute of Orthopedics
San Luis 2534, Rosario 2000, Santa Fe, Argentina

E-mail address:
gastonslullitel@gmail.com

Metatarsalgia
Assessment Algorithm and Decision Making

Valeria Lopez, MD*, Gastón Slullitel, MD

KEYWORDS

• Metatarsalgia • Evaluation algorithm • Treatment • Metatarsal pain

KEY POINTS

• Metatarsalgia should be recognized as a complex isolated entity rather than just a symptom.
• A thorough understanding of the multiple potential causal factors is essential to ensure selection of the optimal treatment.
• General and local conditions can be divided according the location into knee/leg, ankle/hindfoot, and foot. In addition, they can be classified into static and dynamic factors.

INTRODUCTION

Metatarsalgia is typically defined as pain in the forefoot under 1 or more metatarsal heads. This perspective is limited to perceiving metatarsalgia only as a symptom associated with first ray disorders. However, it is necessary to recognize it as a complex and isolated entity.

Historically, metatarsalgia was approached as a forefoot condition, most often associated with hallux valgus. Consequently, surgical treatments were limited to that anatomic zone, disregarding more proximal structures that are now recognized as potential causal factors in the development of metatarsalgia.

In order to assess this entity properly, it is necessary to consider anatomic and biomechanical factors, as well as general and local conditions of the affected patients.

A thorough understanding of the multiple potential causal factors is essential to ensure selection of the optimal treatment.

This article takes a comprehensive approach to metatarsalgia, discussing complete clinical assessment as well as outlining a general treatment algorithm.

Disclosure: The authors have nothing to disclose regarding this publication.
Department of Foot and Ankle Surgery, J Slullitel Institute of Orthopaedics, San Luis 2534, Rosario 2000, Santa Fe, Argentina
* Corresponding author.
E-mail address: vlastegiano@gmail.com

Foot Ankle Clin N Am 24 (2019) 561–569
https://doi.org/10.1016/j.fcl.2019.08.006
1083-7515/19/© 2019 Elsevier Inc. All rights reserved.

ANATOMY

The lesser metatarsal head and the proximal phalanx of the toe are the bony structures that constitute the metatarsophalangeal (MTP) joint. The soft tissues on the dorsum of the MTP joint include the joint capsule and the tendons of extensor digitorum longus and extensor digitorum brevis. The proper and accessory collateral ligaments form the medial and lateral walls, and the plantar plate forms the plantar border of the MTP joint. The flexor digitorum longus (FDL) and flexor digitorum brevis tendons lie on the plantar surface of the plantar plate.[1]

The metatarsal heads are aligned along a harmonious curve in the frontal plane. During weight bearing, the 5 metatarsal heads are at the same distance from the ground. In the sagittal plane, the declination angle decreases from M1 (20°) to M5 (5°). The metatarsals are connected by the transverse intermetatarsal ligament and, therefore, act together as a single functional unit. At the MTP joints, the soft tissues are strengthened by fibrocartilaginous plantar plates, which are functional weight-bearing structures that prevent dorsal dislocation of P1.[2]

BIOMECHANICS

Abnormal biomechanics in the gait cycle can result in metatarsal pain and are identified in the different stages of the gait cycle.

During the swing phase, normal ankle dorsiflexion (20°) is needed for foot clearance, with the tibialis anterior muscle providing the greatest dorsiflexion force. The inability to achieve normal dorsiflexion can be caused by a weak tibialis anterior, Achilles tightness, or other anatomic and biomechanical abnormalities (ie, hind foot varus, cavus foot, and anterior tibiotalar impingement). This over-recruitment of lesser toe extensors can significantly contribute to MTP joint disorders by moving the fat pad distally.[3]

The stance phase is further subdivided into 3 different rocker phases. In the first rocker, the heel acts as a fulcrum, and metatarsalgia in this scenario occurs because of congenital deformity, cavus foot, or a tight heel cord. Afterward, the ankle acts as the second rocker. During this stage the foot remains flat on the ground; however, limited ankle motion and excessively plantarflexed lesser metatarsals may produce second rocker metatarsalgia. In addition, during the third rocker stage, the MTP dorsiflexes while the forefoot is in contact with the ground. Typically, an excessive lesser metatarsal length may cause metatarsalgia, being the most common form throughout the gait cycle.[3]

It is also important to appraise another biomechanical structure: the subtalar joint (STJ). During normal gait, pronation of the STJ converts the foot into a shock-absorbing structure. In supination during the second and third rockers of gait, the foot is converted into a rigid lever, which provides an optimal mechanical efficiency for pushing off. These two physiologic movements (pronation and supination) may become excessive in pathologic conditions (pes planus and pes cavus, respectively) becoming an causal factor in the development of metatarsalgia.

CAUSAL FACTORS

The causal factors of metatarsalgia are classically divided into 3 groups: primary, secondary, and iatrogenic after forefoot surgery[4]:

- Primary metatarsalgia is caused by anatomic characteristics of the metatarsals that affect their relations to one another and to the rest of the foot (eg, excessive M2 or M3 length).

- Secondary metatarsalgia is caused by conditions that increase metatarsal loading via indirect mechanisms (eg, gastrocnemius shortening).
- Iatrogenic metatarsalgia may be the result of a reconstructive procedure on the forefoot (eg, hallux valgus surgery).

However, the authors consider that this classification should be expanded, and potential causal factors need to be categorized into general and local. **Table 1** summarizes our approach to identifying the associated components (see **Table 1**).

General factors include a variety of patient conditions or habits: overweight, maladies such as rheumatoid arthritis, shoe type, hours per day on their feet, and physical activity. It is important to identify these general factors because patients can improve with good advice (eg, losing weight) or changing their habits (eg, shoe type or training routine).

Local conditions can be divided according to the location into knee/leg, ankle/hindfoot, and foot. In addition, they can be classified into static and dynamic factors (**Figs. 1** and **2**).

CLINICAL ASSESSMENT

It is important to perform a complete history and physical examination. The first step is to determine whether metatarsalgia is a primary disorder or secondary to previous trauma or surgery, as well as to rule out diabetes, neuropathy and so forth.

Malalignment of the lower limb and/or foot should be investigated with the patient standing. Genu valgum and varus must be noted. The overall shape of the foot (eg, pes planus or pes cavus) should be described in detail. It is important to assess the midfoot pronation/supination in order to identify subtle cavus foot. Leg length discrepancy should also be noted. Deformities should be classified as reducible or fixed as well. A gait analysis is essential, and patients must be observed walking in bare feet in order to identify different pathologic gait patterns, such as a weak tibialis anterior with FDL over-recruitment, or a supinated gait in patients with hallux rigidus.

Patients are examined in the seated position. It is necessary to identify the point of maximal tenderness. Although not proved, for many years the authors observed a possible correlation between the pain site and the biomechanical impairment: pain in second rocker cases should be expected in the plantar aspect of metatarsal head, whereas in third rocker cases the pain is located more distally.

Table 1
Evaluation of associated factors in patients with metatarsalgia

	Leg	Ankle/Hindfoot	Foot
Static	Genu varum Genu valgum	Ankle equinus	Nonharmonic formulas Forefoot equinus Metatarsus adductus Intraarticular disorders
Dynamic	Gastrocnemius contracture	Limit to dorsiflexion Flat foot Cavus foot Muscle imbalances	First ray disorders Lesser MTPJ instability

Abbreviation: MTPJ, MTP joint.

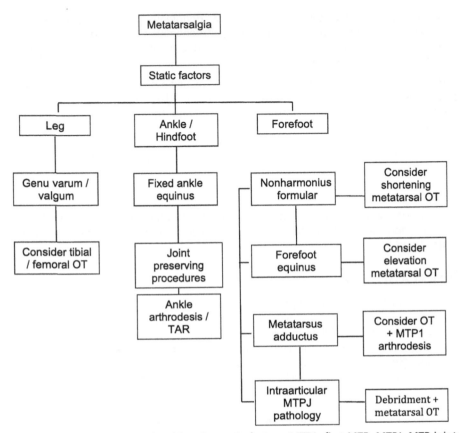

Fig. 1. Proposed treatment algorithm for static factors. MTP1, first MTP; MTPJ, MTP joint; OT, osteotomy; TAR, total ankle replacement.

Inspection of the foot for ulcerations and/or calluses under the metatarsal heads is performed. Keratosis may be localized under a particular metatarsal (second rocker) or may be more diffuse (third rocker) (**Fig. 3**). Nevertheless, many patients have painless keratosis, which should be perceived as an emerging biomechanical imbalance that probably needs to be addressed (eg, stretching exercises and insoles). Surgical treatment is not warranted in this group of patients.

Fat pad atrophy should be identified if present. The forefoot should be examined for hallux valgus, hallux rigidus, or hallux varus, because they can cause a transfer metatarsalgia. Dorsal dislocation or anteroposterior instability (drawer sign) of an MTP joint indicates damage to the plantar plate, and must be checked.[5]

In addition to visual inspection, a neurovascular examination is performed because Morton neuroma is a frequent differential diagnosis.[6] It is necessary to be careful to differentiate a Morton neuroma from mechanical pain, and also to remember that both diagnoses can be made in the same patient.

Passive ranges of motion of the ankle, subtalar joint, and midfoot joint should be recorded. The most important dynamic factor to assess in the supine position consists of performing the maneuvers described by Silfversköld to detect tightness of the gastrocnemius muscles, either alone or in combination with the soleus muscle.[7]

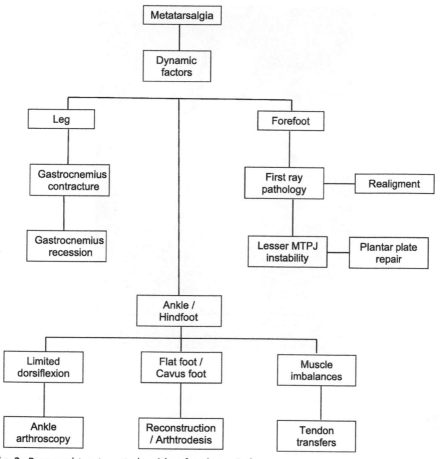

Fig. 2. Proposed treatment algorithm for dynamic factors.

This assessment should be performed in STJ inversion because it reflects the real gastrocnemius tightness.[8]

IMAGING

The radiological examination includes standard weight-bearing radiographs of both feet and ankles. It is also important to add a hindfoot view in order to thoroughly assess the varus/valgus hindfoot alignment. Two available options are the Saltzmann view and the so-called long view.

In foot radiographs clinicians must take note of the presence of first ray disorder (eg, hallux valgus, hallux varus, or hallux rigidus). The length and declination of the lesser metatarsals should also be observed. Metatarsus adductus is a frequent causal factor, and a careful analysis is necessary to avoid underdiagnosing the mild and moderate cases.

The metatarsal heads are normally seen as a curved parabola that has been quantified by Maestro and colleagues,[9] who differentiated several forefoot morphotypes. The relative length of each metatarsal is determined by drawing a line perpendicular to the axis of the foot that runs from the lateral sesamoid to the

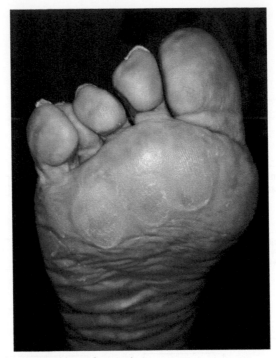

Fig. 3. Second rocker–related hyperkeratosis.

M4 head. Then it is necessary to measure the distances (in millimeters) from each metatarsal head to this line. Three nonharmonious morphotypes can be identified:

- Long M2-M3 morphotype
- M4-M5 hypoplasia
- Long M1 morphotype

Weight-bearing computed tomography provides invaluable information regarding sagittal slope of the lesser metatarsals, enhancing the three-dimensional perspective of the bony components of the deformity.[10]

Ultrasonography and MRI can contribute to the diagnosis of Morton neuroma, intermetatarsal bursitis, flexor tenosynovitis, or a plantar plate lesion.

TREATMENT ALGORITHM

The first-line treatment is conservative, and surgery should be considered only when conservative treatment fails for at least 6 months.

The first step is to address the general factors (eg, losing weight, gastrocnemius stretching program, shoe modifications) as well as to try local measures (eg, insoles) in order to relieve pain. Note that most patients improve with conservative treatment. Nevertheless, there is little high-level evidence (level I) to support the efficacy of conservative treatment of metatarsalgia[11,12]

Once conservative treatment has failed, surgical treatment is indicated. It is difficult to draw a simple treatment algorithm, because each patient is different from the others. As with any condition, management is tailored to the cause or causes.

At this point it is therefore necessary to review all the causal factors that affect the patient, and make a careful preoperative plan that includes all these factors.

Knee/Leg

Clinicians should start by assessing proximal disorders (knee/leg). If the patient has a genu varus that overloads de fourth and fifth metatarsals, a proximal tibial osteotomy is needed to restore the leg alignment. In contrast, if a genu valgum is present, and the overload affects the medial metatarsals, a distal femoral osteotomy might be considered for the same purpose.

If there is a gastrocnemius shortening, a gastrocnemius recession must be performed. There are different techniques that are discussed in Gastón Slullitel and Juan Pablo Calvi's article, "Gastrocnemius Recession in the Setting of Metatarsalgia: The Baumann Procedure," in this issue. If the shortening also affects the soleus muscle, an Achilles tendon lengthening (ATL) is needed.

Ankle/Hindfoot

If there is limited ankle dorsiflexion, anterior ankle impingement may be the diagnosis. Anterior ankle arthroscopy is performed in order to remove the anterior tibial and talar osteophytes. This procedure mechanically decompresses the anterior ankle joint and eases the pain. Cases with more severe arthritis and rigid deformities may need an ankle replacement (with ATL) or an ankle arthrodesis in order to restore the sagittal imbalance.

Pes cavus may also be the causal factor. If so, soft tissue procedures (plantar fascia lengthening), different osteotomies (calcaneal, first metatarsal, distal tibia), as well as some tendon transfers (posterior tibial tendon to the dorsum, peroneus longus to brevis) must be included in order to restore the foot balance. In severe cases, triple arthrodesis is necessary to realign the foot. In this scenario (pes cavus), it is important to correct the whole foot in order to avoid the common mistake of performing only forefoot procedures.

Pes planus frequently also needs to be corrected. Typically, a calcaneal osteotomy is needed (medializing osteotomy or lateral column lengthening) associated with soft tissue procedures (posterior tibial tendon debridement and/or FDL or FHL tendon transfers). It is important to include ATL or gastrocnemius recession, because this is a key factor in these patients. Severe cases may also need a triple arthrodesis.

In addition, a steppage deformity can follow a neurologic disorder. This equinus deformity can cause metatarsal pain that may need a surgical solution. In this scenario a posterior tibial tendon transfer may solve the problem. It is also important to consider a gastrocnemius or Achilles lengthening in order to balance the ankle in the sagittal plane.

Foot

If a first ray disorder is identified (eg, hallux valgus, hallux varus, hallux rigidus) it must be corrected. This correction can be achieved via different osteotomies, soft tissue procedures, or MTP joint arthrodesis. Restoring the function of the first ray unloads the lesser metatarsals, and although this concept, so-called first ray insufficiency, is accepted worldwide, there is a lack of evidence that supports it.[13] Therefore, it should not be oversized, and first ray procedures should be performed only in order to alleviate metatarsal pain. The most frequent scenario is that many concurrent procedures need to be performed because patients usually have a variety of causal factors.

The anteroposterior weight-bearing radiograph serves to assess the relative positions of the metatarsal heads along a harmonious or disharmonious curve. If a disharmonious Maestro curve is observed, Weil osteotomies must be performed in order to restore a normal metatarsal parabola.

If sagittal imbalance is identified, a triple Maceira osteotomy[4] is necessary to address this deformity. If the metatarsal slope is more severe (eg, forefoot equinus or pes cavus), proximal osteotomies are needed (eg, Barouk-Rippstein-Toullec osteotomy-type basal osteotomies).

In patients with MTP joint instability, a plantar plate repair or a tendon transfer (flexor to extensor) can be performed in combination with arthroplasty or arthrodesis of the proximal interphalangeal and/or distal interphalangeal joints.

Metatarsus adductus is a difficult problem to solve. The mainly mild deformities constitute a diagnostic challenge, and are frequently misdiagnosed, which is one of the main causes of hallux valgus surgery failure. In these cases, clinicians must obtain a proper first ray alignment and also perform lesser metatarsal osteotomies[13] to realign the forefoot adequately.

Although not common, degenerative joint disease (eg, Freiberg disease) may be diagnosed. In these cases, different scenarios may require simple debridement, metatarsal osteotomies, and/or resection arthroplasty. It is desirable to try a joint-preserving procedure initially, because these patients often require revision surgeries.

Another important factor, lesser toe deformities (claw toes, hammer toes, and mallet toes), should be properly fixed in order to unload MTP joints.

SUMMARY

Metatarsalgia can be a considerable source of pain and dysfunction. Obtaining a careful history and performing a focused examination helps identify the causal factors that are involved. In order to assess this entity properly, it is necessary to consider anatomic and biomechanical factors, as well as general and local conditions of the affected patients. A thorough understanding of the multiple causal factors is essential to ensure selection of the optimal treatment.

REFERENCES

1. Finney FT, Cata E, Holmes JR, et al. Anatomy and physiology of the lesser metatarsophalangeal joints. Foot Ankle Clin 2018;23(1):1–7.
2. Besse JL. Metatarsalgia. Orthop Traumatol Surg Res 2017;103(1S):S29–39 [Review].
3. Federer AE, Tainter DM, Adams SB, et al. Conservative management of metatarsalgia and lesser toe deformities. Foot Ankle Clin 2018;23(1):9–20 [Review].
4. Espinosa N, Brodsky JW, Maceira E. Metatarsalgia. J Am Acad Orthop Surg 2010;18(8):474–85 [Review].
5. Nery C, Coughlin MJ, Baumfeld D, et al. Prospective evaluation of protocol for surgical treatment of lesser MTP joint plantar plate tears. Foot Ankle Int 2014; 35(9):876–85.
6. DiPreta JA. Metatarsalgia, lesser toe deformities, and associated disorders of the forefoot. Med Clin North Am 2014;98(2):233–51.
7. Symeonidis P. The Silfverskiöld Test. Foot Ankle Int 2014;35(8):838.
8. Cortina RE, Morris BL, Vopat BG. Gastrocnemius recession for metatarsalgia. Foot Ankle Clin 2018;23(1):57–68 [Review].
9. Maestro M, Besse JL, Ragusa M, et al. Forefoot morphotype study and planning method for forefoot osteotomy. Foot Ankle Clin 2003;8(4):695–710 [Review].

10. Cheung ZB, Myerson MS, Tracey J, et al. Weightbearing CT scan assessment of foot alignment in patients with hallux rigidus. Foot Ankle Int 2018;39(1): 67–74.
11. Espinosa N, Maceira E, Myerson MS. Current concept review: metatarsalgia. Foot Ankle Int 2008;29(8):871–9 [Review].
12. Slullitel G, López V, Calvi JP, et al. Effect of first ray insufficiency and metatarsal index on metatarsalgia in hallux valgus. Foot Ankle Int 2016;37(3):300–6.
13. Aiyer AA, Shariff R, Ying L, et al. Prevalence of metatarsus adductus in patients undergoing hallux valgus surgery. Foot Ankle Int 2014;35(12):1292–7.

Mechanical Basis of Metatarsalgia

Ernesto Maceira, MD[a], Manuel Monteagudo, MD[b,*]

KEYWORDS

• Metatarsalgia • Biomechanics • Gait • Metatarsal osteotomy • Forefoot

KEY POINTS

- Identification and hierarchization of the mechanical impairments involved in each case is critical in order to eliminate pain and restore foot function as much as possible.
- Functional or anatomic equinus is important during the second and the early third rocker but not at the late propulsive phase.
- Metatarsal length is important in third-rocker disorders but not in second-rocker overload.
- Patients may present with combined second-rocker and third-rocker disorder at a given ray or at different rays.
- There are several things that should not be done and that may be useful in the surgical planning of mechanical metatarsalgia: do not shorten a metatarsal with evidence of second-rocker overload (second-rocker keratosis, extensor over-recruitment), otherwise overloading will persist and the toe will develop additional dorsiflexion contracture; do not elevate a metatarsal with evidence of third-rocker overload (third-rocker keratosis, metacarpophalangeal joint instability), otherwise a central ray insufficiency syndrome may develop with second-rocker overload at the neighboring rays; do not lengthen the gastrocnemius in the absence of gastrocnemius-dependent equinus, as is the case in pure third-rocker disorder.

 Video content accompanies this article at http://www.foot.theclinics.com.

INTRODUCTION: PREVIOUS THEORIES, THE 3 FOOT ROCKERS, AND THE TISSUE STRESS THEORIES

This article deals with the pathogenesis of mechanical metatarsalgia and offers a clinical guide to identifying the primary mechanical impairment responsible for the signs and symptoms that may be present in patients with metatarsalgia.

Disclosure: The authors and their spouses have no relevant professional or financial affiliations.
[a] Orthopaedic Foot and Ankle Unit, Complejo Hospitalario La Mancha Centro, Av de la Constitución 3, 13600 Alcazar de San Juan, Ciudad Real, Spain; [b] Orthopaedic Foot and Ankle Unit, Orthopaedic and Trauma Department, Hospital Universitario Quirónsalud Madrid, Faculty Medicine UEM, Calle Diego de Velázquez 1, Pozuelo de Alarcón, Madrid 28223, Spain
* Corresponding author.
E-mail address: mmontyr@yahoo.com

Foot Ankle Clin N Am 24 (2019) 571–584
https://doi.org/10.1016/j.fcl.2019.08.008

foot.theclinics.com

Because people have limbs instead of wheels, they need a mechanism to simultaneously achieve continuous progression and stable support, and this is provided by the 3-rocker mechanism, first described by Jacqueline Perry.[1] During the stance phase, the tibia of the supporting limb keeps on rotating forward on 3 different rocking axes. In normal conditions the initial contact of the foot takes place at the heel, on which the tibia rotates forward until the forefoot contacts the ground (first rocker or heel rocker). Once the foot is plantigrade on the ground, the tibia rotates on the talus (second rocker or ankle rocker; the supporting limb must be functionally long to allow opposite limb clearance) and, when the body center of mass lies anterior with respect to the foot, the tibia rotates on the metatarsophalangeal break line (third rocker or forefoot rocker). The foot-ground contact pattern is different in each rocker (**Fig. 1**): during the first rocker (10% of the gait cycle), just the heel contacts the ground; during the second rocker (20% of the gait cycle), although the supporting limb is solely responsible for the body-weight support, the foot shows the most stable contact pattern, the plantigrade support.[1] The third-rocker or propulsive phase accounts for 30% of the gait cycle and the foot-ground contact area is limited to the forefoot, including both the toes and the metatarsal pad.

Mechanical metatarsalgia is assumed to be a symptom caused by tissue stress (both bony and soft tissue stress), which in turn is produced by mechanical impairments.[2] Thus the key to success in management of metatarsalgia is the identification of the main mechanical impairments in a given patient by studying the consequences of stress on the patient's structures and tissues. Apart from pain, tissue stress may also produce deformities and histologic changes, such as keratoses, soft tissue–itis, soft tissue–osis, soft tissue rupture, bony adaptations, bone stress reactions, fractures, and so forth. It is difficult to find the cause in many patients. However, when searching for the main mechanical impairment, it is easier to assess which structures have nothing to do with the condition. Has metatarsal length anything to do in this particular patient? If not, do not focus the treatment on metatarsal length modification.

TYPES OF MECHANICAL METATARSALGIA: PROPULSIVE VERSUS NONPROPULSIVE

Propulsive metatarsalgia is produced during the third rocker, whereas nonpropulsive metatarsalgia is the result of mechanical impairments acting during any other phase of the gait cycle.[3] During the swing phase and the first rocker, the forefoot does not support weight, but it is exposed to deforming forces such as extensor over-recruitment, a compensatory mechanism for equinism.

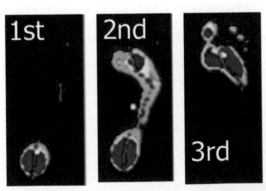

Fig. 1. Interface contact patterns during the first, second, and third rockers of gait.

Propulsive metatarsalgia is caused by stress during the propulsive phase (third rocker) (**Fig. 2**). The ground contact pattern includes the toes and the metatarsal eminence or metatarsal pad. The structures involved are the soft tissues located plantar and distal to the metatarsal head (skin, plantar plates) and the bones (axial compression of the metatarsals). Metatarsal length, particularly the relative overall length of the 5 metatarsals, is crucial to provide adequate loading distribution among all metatarsals, avoiding stress concentration (**Fig. 3**). The foot is placed vertical on the plantar metatarsal pad, transmitting the body weight mainly along the tibia, talus, navicular, and the 3 medial rays (this is referred to as the talar foot or medial column).[4] Adduction of the first metatarsal during the third rocker may behave as an anatomically short metatarsal; in both cases, third-rocker tissue stress lesions may be present in the lesser rays.

Nonpropulsive metatarsalgia is produced in any phase other than the third rocker, including the swing phase, the first rocker, and the second rocker. During the second rocker, the foot must be plantigrade on the ground. During plantigrade support, the forefoot bears external dorsiflexing moments produced by ground reaction forces and inertial parameters. During midstance support, the body weight is distributed toward the heel and the forefoot, thus increasing the interface area with the ground. Metatarsal length is not as relevant as it is during the third rocker. Anatomic and/or functional inclination of the metatarsals is crucial to ensure adequate load distribution underneath every metatarsal head.[3] Soft tissues anatomically located strictly plantar to the corresponding head/s experience compressive stresses during this phase. The plantar plate is less damaged by mechanical stress during the second rocker when compared with the third rocker (**Fig. 4**). Metatarsals are exposed to dorsiflexing moments, but there is another force that can stress tissues in nonpropulsive

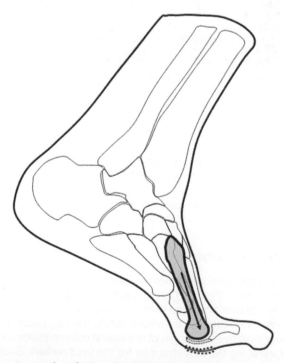

Fig. 2. Tissue stress generation during the third rocker.

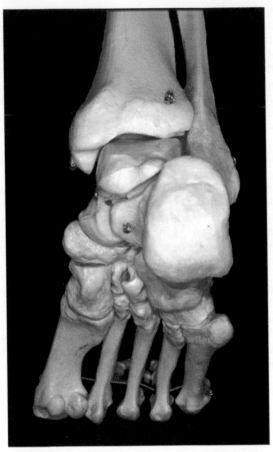

Fig. 3. At the end of the third rocker, the relative length among metatarsals is important for the generation of metatarsalgia.

metatarsalgia: extensor tendon over-recruitment.[3] In normal conditions, the extensor digitorum longus helps the tibialis anterior muscle in producing ankle dorsiflexion moments during the swing phase and the first rocker. As soon as the forefoot contacts the ground, they both should end their action (Video 1).[5] Dorsiflexion of the toes during part of the second rocker indicates an additional dorsiflexing moment at the ankle that is needed in order to compensate for the increased plantarflexor moments at the ankle joint (Video 2).[3]

PATTERNS OF PLANTAR KERATOSES

Second-rocker (nonpropulsive) keratoses are located strictly plantar to the head of the corresponding metatarsals (**Fig. 5**). During the second rocker, the leg externally rotates over the ankle-hindfoot universal joint (peritalar complex). Transverse plane motion is produced on the hindfoot to externally rotate the leg, placing the origin of the medial column (talar foot) over the origin of the lateral column (calcaneal foot), thus supinating the foot (preparing the foot structure for the third rocker). Because during this rocker there is no rotating effect between the foot and the ground, each keratosis is

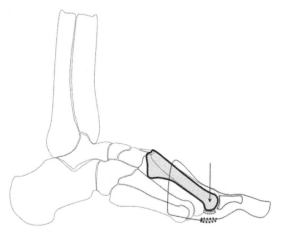

Fig. 4. Tissue stress generation during the second rocker. Metatarsal length is not relevant during this phase. During the second rocker, anatomic or functional inclination of the metatarsals is important for the generation of metatarsalgia.

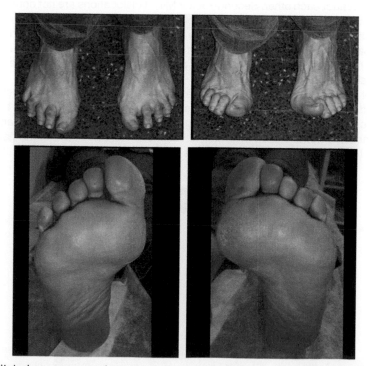

Fig. 5. Clinical appearance of second-rocker (nonpropulsive) metatarsalgia in the patient shown in Video 2. The patient is unable to lift the forefoot standing on the heels. Tibialis anterior muscle is normal in function but cannot cope with the increased plantarflexor moment provided by the short elastic component of the gastrocnemius. Note second-rocker keratoses on the sole of the feet.

limited to its corresponding metatarsal, with no tendency to join to neighboring lesions.

In contrast, the main morphologic feature of third-rocker keratoses is their distal extension toward the base of the corresponding toes. They are located plantodistal to the corresponding metatarsal heads. Because during the third rocker the foot rotates externally on the ground, third-rocker keratoses frequently fuse with neighboring keratoses so a single rounded broad keratosis may appear, making it difficult to assess which part of it corresponds to each of the metatarsals involved (**Fig. 6**).[3]

At the fifth metatarsal, both second-rocker and third-rocker keratoses may present as well. Second-rocker keratoses, strictly plantar to the fifth metatarsal head, are related to hindfoot varus. They may appear together with plantar keratosis underneath the metatarsal base. Third-rocker keratoses at the anterolateral margin of the foot are produced by foot supination that is generated to compensate for the lack of dorsiflexion of the first metatarsophalangeal joint during the propulsive phase.

PATTERNS OF METATARSOPHALANGEAL JOINT DISLOCATION

The plantar plate is loaded during the third rocker while the metatarsal bone is vertical on the ground transmitting axial compressive forces. Chronic overloading of the plantar plate may eventually rupture it, thus allowing the base of the phalanx to dislocate dorsally. Third-rocker metatarsophalangeal joint (MTPJ) dislocations are complete dislocations because the articular surfaces of the phalanx and the metatarsal no longer contact each other. Second-rocker MTPJ dislocations are not complete dislocations but subluxations, because one of the articular surfaces (the proximal articular surface of the proximal phalanx) keeps contact with the other bone (metatarsal). In the second-rocker dislocation, the proximal phalanx of the toe remains erect, vertical on the metatarsal head. The plantar plate is not injured in pure second-rocker dislocations.[3]

Several patients may present with stigmata of both types of mechanical metatarsalgia (mixed metatarsalgia), making those cases difficult to analyze. During the transition from second to third rocker, the supporting limb is required to dorsiflex the ankle and extend the knee at the same time, making this instant (around 50% of the gait cycle) the peak tensioning moment of the Achilles-calcaneus-plantar system (**Fig. 7**). Some

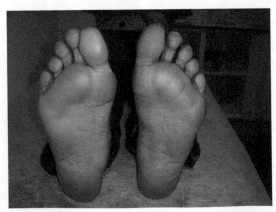

Fig. 6. Clinical appearance of third-rocker (propulsive) keratosis. Note the distal extension of the keratosis toward the base of the toes. Both the second and third metatarsals contribute to the formation of a big, rounded keratosis.

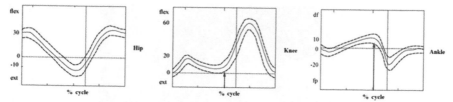

Fig. 7. At around 50% of the gait cycle, at the transition from the second to the third rocker, the ankle needs to dorsiflex and the knee must be extended at the same time, so gastrocnemius retraction is particularly harmful at this point. The normal kinematic record of the hip (*left*), knee (*middle*), and ankle joint (*right*). Both maximal knee extension and ankle dorsiflexion occur together at 50% of the gait cycle.

brainstorming is needed to clear up the scenario and make some sense in the pathogenesis of any given case of metatarsalgia. Increased stress during the transition from the second to the third rocker may result in mixed metatarsalgia with stigmata of both rockers.

MORPHOLOGIC FEATURES INDICATING MECHANICAL ADAPTATION

Sometimes mechanical impairments are suggested by certain surface anatomy peculiarities.

The dorsal bump at the dorsum of the first cuneometatarsal joint is commonly associated with a short first metatarsal. It seems to be the result of an adaptation process to provide first metatarsal head support during static stance phase of gait. Osteoarthritic changes may or may not be present. Sometimes it is just the flexed position of the first metatarsal with respect to the medial cuneiform that causes the joint to protrude dorsally. The first and second metatarsals usually show the same inclination angle with respect to the ground plane. This angle can be seen in the lateral view of a weight-bearing radiograph (the dorsal cortices of their diaphyses are parallel to each other). In the presence of a short first metatarsal, its head is not able to contact the ground during plantigrade support unless increased plantarflexion of the first metatarsal is achieved. The authors believe the dorsal cuneometatarsal bump is the result of osseous adaptation to compensate for M1 shortness, with a plantarflexed first tarsometatarsal joint with or without osteoarthritis changes (**Fig. 8**).

Frequently, functional hallux limitus/rigidus presents with a typical spoonlike shape of the first ray because the first metatarsal bone is dorsiflexed and the first MTPJ is plantarflexed, whereas the interphalangeal joint of the first toe is dorsiflexed (**Fig. 9**). In addition, the plantar skin underneath the first metatarsal head shows no signs of wearing, whereas the skin under the second metatarsal head may present with a second-rocker keratosis and the fifth ray may show a third-rocker keratosis. Functional hallux limitus/rigidus must be examined with a specific test with dorsiflexion of the first toe while simulating loading and unloading conditions (see Videos 1 and 2; Video 3).

Divergence of the second and third toes in static stance is usually part of a second-space syndrome (see nerve entrapments at the forefoot, later in the text) (**Fig. 10**). In our experience, whenever the second toe is adducted, distal protrusion of the second metatarsal with respect to the first and/or the third metatarsal is also present (but not vice versa). Overlapping second toe over the hallux develops when there is adduction of the second toe together with limited dorsiflexion of the hallux.

Stress on the metatarsal bones is also different during the second and third rocker. During the third rocker, the metatarsal is axially loaded, supporting axial compression

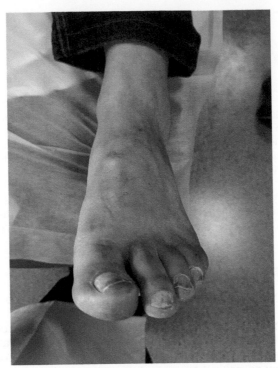

Fig. 8. In some patients with a short first metatarsal, an increase of the inclination angle of the bone may provide for adequate ground contact of the first metatarsal head during plantigrade support. As a result, the first cuneiform-metatarsal joint may show a dorsal bump, with or without osteoarthritis changes on the radiograph.

all along its structure. In the case of stress concentration on a metatarsal, it fails where bony tissue is less resistant to compression; that is, at the metatarsal head, where the bone is cancellous, not compact. Freiberg disease is the consequence of increased stress during the third rocker of gait. A distal compression fracture develops, thus shortening the metatarsal up to the point of an ideal metatarsal parabola. The stress supported by the metatarsals during the second rocker produces dorsiflexory moments to the bone, creating compression at the dorsal cortex and distraction at the plantar cortex. Bony failure occurs at the point where the dorsiflexory gradient and bone thickness combined exceed the elastic tension module of compact bone at the plantar cortex, resulting in a dorsiflexory stress fracture (**Fig. 11**).

Nerve entrapment may take place at the distal intermetatarsal spaces. Chronic repeated microtrauma may produce nerve enlargement and simulate a neoplastic formation that, in turn, may worsen neural compression. Compression of the third common digital nerve may take place in a mechanically normal foot for anatomic reasons, such as the connection of the medial plantar and lateral plantar nerve branches, and mechanical reasons, such as the different range of motion of the third and fourth metatarsal bones on the sagittal plane.[4] Both at the beginning and at the end of the second rocker, shearing stress may occur at the third space in a healthy, normal-functioning foot. At the beginning of the third rocker, nerve entrapment may take place between the plantar soft tissues of the space and the deep transverse intermetatarsal ligament dorsally. The effect worsens if the nerve is enlarged, producing a vicious-circle effect.

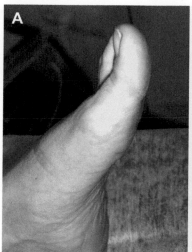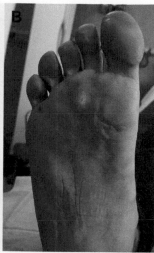

Fig. 9. Clinical signs of forefoot disorders. (*A*) Spoonlike first ray in functional hallux limitus-rigidus. It is the consequence of an elevated first metatarsal head together with first MTPJ plantarflexion and interphalangeal joint dorsiflexion. A keratosis usually develops at the plantar aspect of the interphalangeal joint and there is no evidence of skin wear underneath the first metatarsal head. (*B*) Second-rocker keratosis may develop at the middle metatarsal heads, particularly under the second metatarsal. Although an exostosis will eventually develop at the first metatarsal head, it may present no osteoarthritic changes at initial stages.

However, in the second space, there is no difference in the sagittal range of motion of the second and third metatarsals. The second-space syndrome, first mentioned by Serré and André as Viladot describes in his book *Patología del Antepié* [Forefoot Pathology] (1974), is a group of signs and symptoms, including the divergence of the second and third toes, with the second adducted on bipedal support (may not diverge in the unloaded foot), and neuritic symptoms similar to those experienced in Morton neuroma of the third space[6] (see **Fig. 10**). Patients with second-space syndrome frequently present with a third-rocker keratosis. The authors have almost always found some amount of second metatarsal protrusion with respect to the first and/or the third metatarsals and we consider it a propulsive lesion, although we cannot explain why the second toe adducts and the second metatarsal head deviates laterally on the weight-bearing radiographs. This situation produces compression stress on the soft tissues in the second metatarsal space. A medial-sliding Weil osteotomy is indicated in these patients. Common digital nerve compression at the second space is usually produced by transverse compression between the second and third metatarsal heads, and this occurs when the second toe is medially deviated. As stated earlier, adduction of the second toe usually develops when the second metatarsal is longer than it should be with respect to the first and/or the third metatarsals in relation to the ideal metatarsal parabola (see **Fig. 10**). With a different pathogenesis, Morton neuropathy of the third metatarsal space occurs in a normofunctioning foot just by the difference in sagittal plane range of motion between the lateral cuneometatarsal joint and the cuboid–fourth metatarsal joint. Entrapment of the second common digital nerve requires an important mechanical impairment to explain repeated trauma to the nerve, and nerve enlargement must be secondary to cyclic trauma. Clinicians should look for traumatic stress in these patients and there is almost always a mechanical explanation

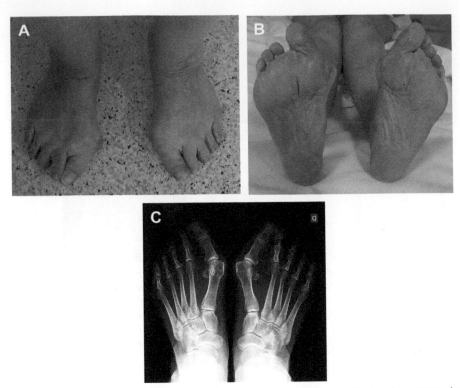

Fig. 10. Second-space syndrome. (*A*) Clinical appearance during static standing. Note the divergence of the second and third toes, which may be unnoticed in the unloaded foot. (*B*) The plantar surface may show stigmata of third-rocker keratosis. (*C*) Weight-bearing radiographs show divergence of the toes, relative protrusion of the second metatarsal with respect to the first and/or the third metatarsal bones, and narrowing of the second intermetatarsal space caused by abduction of the second metatarsal.

for any metatarsal pain. Clinical examination sheds light on the mechanical cause of metatarsalgia.

CLINICAL EXAMINATION OF PATIENTS WITH METATARSALGIA

Plantar keratoses, when present, are clues to the kind of stress that is responsible for the clinical condition of each patient. The presence of extensor over-recruitment and/ or the inability for the patient to walk on the heels, or even the inability to stand on the heels, should lead clinicians to suspect that there is some kind of subclinical equinus. The Silfverskiöld test help in assessing whether gastrocnemius retraction is the only mechanism responsible for the equinus (positive test) or whether there is something else producing it (negative test; no increase in ankle dorsiflexion when the knee is flexed) (Video 4).[7] If there is equinus and ankle dorsiflexion does not improve when flexing the knee, look for joint blockage or soleus involvement. Barouk and Barouk[8] combined the functional hallux limitus/rigidus test and the Silfverskiöld test to determine whether a given case of functional hallux limitus/rigidus was directly related to gastrocnemius retraction. When there is direct responsibility of the gastrocnemius in a patient with functional hallux limitus/rigidus, the flexor hallucis longus test is

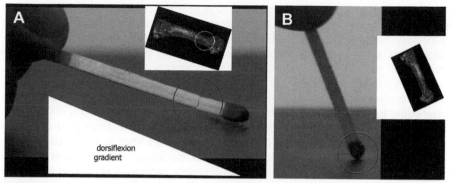

Fig. 11. Metatarsal bony stress. (*A*) During the second rocker, the metatarsals have to bear dorsiflexor moments. The moment is greater at the proximal end of the bone and smaller at the distal end (dorsiflexion moment is null at the center of the metatarsal head and increases toward the proximal end because of the dorsiflexing moment arm). Failure of the bone takes place at the point where the combination of bone geometry and moment arm exceeds the tensile resistance of cortical bone located at the metatarsal neck where the bone is thinner. A dorsiflexion fracture occurs, which is known as stress fracture or Deutschländer fracture. (*B*) During the third rocker, the metatarsal bone is vertical on the ground, supporting axial compression all along its length. The point of failure is where bone structure is weaker to compression; this is at the metatarsal head, which is made out of cancellous bone instead of the compact bone of the diaphysis. This fracture is also a stress fracture, but it is called Freiberg disease. Blood flow to the distal end of the metatarsal may be interrupted by this type of stress compression fracture.

pathologic with the knee extended, but shows normal kinetics when the knee is flexed (Video 5).

A typical case of third-rocker metatarsalgia would be a patient with chronic pain around the metatarsophalangeal break line. The first metatarsal is slightly shorter than the second metatarsal, there is mild clinical deformity, but weight-bearing dorsoplantar foot radiograph shows mild adduction of the first metatarsal bone with mild hallux valgus deformity. The ideal metatarsal parabola may be defined as that metatarsal formula with less active requirement to provide the forefoot with the best support distribution along all of the metatarsal heads, as described by Viladot,[4] Leliévre and Leliévre,[9] and Maestro.[10,11] The metatarsophalangeal break line represents a parabola with the first 2 metatarsals being similar in length when observed on weight-bearing radiographs. In the presence of even a mild prominence in the length of one or several metatarsals, and given that loading is repeated more than 3,000,000 times a year (which is the standard number of gait cycles performed by a moderate-activity population), the corresponding metatarsal may end up stressing the plantar plate, which eventually either ruptures or detaches from the base of the corresponding toe.[12] After a period of swelling and increasing pain, the pain disappears for some time but the toe is lifted up and gets shorter and shorter. The patient then experiences metatarsalgia of varying intensity. The second toe is dislocated dorsally and looks shortened and parallel to the ground but is unable to purchase the ground. Sometime later, second-rocker keratoses clearly develop underneath the heads of the second and third metatarsals within the contour of a previous third-rocker keratosis. Special attention should be paid to the general foot alignment. Mild subtalar protonation may develop almost inadvertently and render symptomatic a foot that was previously healthy.

A typical case of second-rocker metatarsalgia affects a middle-aged patient without any neurologic disorder and with a history of metatarsophalangeal pain, shoe rubbing on the toes, with toe clawing and hardness of the sole of the foot. On clinical examination, there are several independent keratoses strictly plantar to the central metatarsal heads, with toe clawing because of the pulling of the long extensor tendons. The metatarsophalangeal joints are flexible but tend to dorsiflex spontaneously. On visual gait analysis, the toes are moving dorsally even during plantigrade support. The Silfverskiöld test (performed with the foot in subtalar inversion to block any intrinsic foot dorsiflexion) shows increased passive dorsiflexion at the ankle joint when the knee is flexed, compared with the same motion when the knee is extended.

Both cases described earlier include many of the signs and symptoms of third-rocker versus second-rocker metatarsalgia. In some patients it is difficult to identify the main impairments producing the disease. Judicious clinical examination together with weight-bearing radiographs of both feet may provide enough information to assess which kind of mechanical metatarsalgia the patient has, or the clinician might at least be able to rule out those mechanical parameters that have nothing to do with the patient's pain.

RADIOLOGICAL EXAMINATION OF THE WEIGHT-BEARING FOOT

Weight-bearing radiographs should be taken with the patient in bipedal standing support. The dorsoplantar view must be centered and focused between both feet, in order to make the examination repeatable and reliable. The second cuneometatarsal joint must be clearly seen (the joint must show an orthogonal projection). The lateral view should be able to show the tibia perpendicular to the ground. It is difficult to measure (quantify) angles on radiographs, particularly in nonlong bones, such as the talus and calcaneus. However, it is easier to assess whether the medial column is properly aligned or not. Clinicians should be able to visualize a "brochette" made out of the talus, navicular, first cuneiform, and first metatarsal, both in the dorsoplantar and lateral views. The talus and the first metatarsal must be coaxial to each other. The second metatarsal must continue the bisector between the talus and the calcaneus on the dorsoplantar view. The examiner should be able to identify abduction or adduction at the tarsometatarsal or the midtarsal joints (or a combination of both deformities, as occurs in the difficult skewfoot or Z foot). Length measurements on weight-bearing radiographs are reliable. The metatarsal parabola is easy to identify, particularly in the normally hindfoot to forefoot aligned foot with the axis of the second metatarsal as a reference. Maestro[10,11] stated that the center of the lateral sesamoid of the first ray and the center of the fourth metatarsal head should lie at the same level in the dorsoplantar view.

Unlike other investigators, the authors do not measure intermetatarsal angles. It is impossible to measure angles intraoperatively. If there is adduction of the first metatarsal, we quantify (preoperatively and intraoperatively) the lateral displacement required for the first metatarsal head to lie over the sesamoids.

SURGICAL PLANNING OF MECHANICAL METATARSALGIA

In a propulsive/third-rocker metatarsalgia, the authors prefer to measure the amount of shortening required at each of the metatarsals to achieve an ideal metatarsal parabola. In the presence of any metatarsophalangeal propulsive dislocation, the authors redraw a new parabola over the dislocated joint (or the worst of the dislocations). We use a trace drawing on the dorsoplantar weight-bearing radiograph to quantify the amount of shortening required at each metatarsal (**Fig. 12**). Whenever a third-rocker

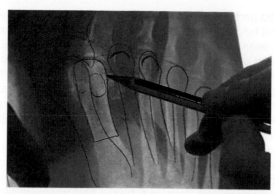

Fig. 12. It is advisable to use a trace drawing on the dorsoplantar weight-bearing radiograph to quantify the amount of shortening required at each metatarsal. Quantification in millimeters (not degrees) in the presurgical planning allows a more reliable surgical procedure and outcome.

dislocation is present, we do not try to replace the toe to its original location, but instead shorten the metatarsal to the point that allows reduction of the dislocation. We then consider the medial and lateral metatarsals to estimate the shortening needed at the nondislocated MTPJs in order to achieve an ideal parabola (**Fig. 13**).[3] For shortenings larger than 2 mm, we use the triple Weil osteotomy rather than the conventional Weil, in order to avoid postoperative stiffness and/or floating toes. We also perform triple Weil osteotomies if we look for a mild elevating effect of the metatarsal (ie, mixed metatarsalgia).

In nonpropulsive/second-rocker metatarsalgia, patients with evidence of extensor over-recruitment do not benefit from metatarsal shortening. They may need gastrocnemius lengthening together with release of the long extensor tendons, with or without transfer of the extensors to the dorsum of the foot in order to increase the internal dorsiflexor moment at the ankle joint. In the presence of gastrocnemius-dependent

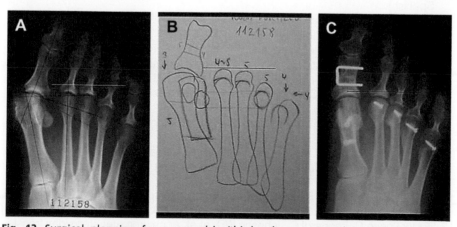

Fig. 13. Surgical planning for a propulsive/third-rocker metatarsalgia. (*A*) Preoperative weight-bearing dorsoplantar radiograph with hallux valgus and index minus. (*B*) Preoperative planning. (*C*) Postoperative weight-bearing dorsoplantar radiograph showing hallux valgus correction and a harmonical metatarsal parabola.

equinus, the authors perform a proximal medial gastrocnemius release in the way Barouk and Barouk did for metatarsalgia.[8] In nonpropulsive MTPJ subluxations (not true dislocations), we release the extensor digitorum longus from the toes. In addition, we reattach the released long extensor tendons to the dorsum of the foot with the use of an anchor or an interference screw if we estimate the internal plantarflexor moment is important, although we have no objective indicators to establish when to perform this procedure. The location for the reattachment of the long extensors is a medial or lateral tarsal bone, depending on whether we want additional inverting or everting moments to act in the patient.

Keeping in mind that metatarsalgia is a symptom, metatarsal pain may be the first symptom of a mayor deformity or impairment at a more proximal location. Clinicians should therefore never forget to check for hindfoot alignment, arch structure, and so forth. An isolated calcaneal osteotomy may be the best treatment of a particular case of metatarsalgia (Video 6). In patients with functional hallux limitus/rigidus, gastrocnemius lengthening together with hindfoot osteotomies and first metatarsal plantarflexion osteotomies may be indicated.[13]

SUPPLEMENTARY DATA

Supplementary data related to this article can be found online at https://doi.org/10.1016/j.fcl.2019.08.008.

REFERENCES

1. Perry J. Gait analysis: normal and pathological function. Thorofare (New Jersey): Slack; 1992.
2. McPoil TG, Hunt GC. Evaluation and management of foot and ankle disorders: present problems and future directions. J Orthop Sports Phys Ther 1995;21(6): 381–8.
3. Espinosa N, Maceira E, Myerson MS. Current concept review: metatarsalgia. Foot Ankle Int 2008;29:871–9.
4. Viladot A. Fifteen lessons on foot pathology. [Quince lecciones sobre patologia del pie]. 2nd edition. Barcelona (Spain): Springer-Verlag Iberica; 2000 [in Spanish].
5. Kirtley C. Clinical gait analysis. Theory and practice. Philadelphia (USA): Churchill Livingstone Elsevier; 2006. ISBN 0 4431 0009 8.
6. Viladot-Pericé A. Patología del antepié. Barcelona: Toray; 1974.
7. Silfverskiöld N. Reduction of the uncrossed two-joints muscles of the leg to one joint muscles in spastic conditions. Acta Chir Scand 1924;56:53.
8. Barouk LS, Barouk P. Compte-rendu symposium gastrocnémien court. Toulouse. Maitrise Orthopédique 2006;159:21–8.
9. Leliévre J, Leliévre JF. Pathology of the foot. [Pathologie du pied]. 5th edition. Paris: Masson; 1981.
10. Maestro M, Augoyard M, Barouk LS, et al. Biomècanique et rèperes radiologiques du sèsamoide latèral de l'hallux par rapport à la palette mètatasienne. Mèd Chir Pied 1995;11-3:145–54.
11. Maestro M, Besse JL, Ragusa M, et al. Forefoot morphotype study and planning method for forefoot osteotomy. Foot Ankle Clin 2003;8:695–710.
12. Tudor-Locke C, Leonardi C, Johnson WD, et al. Accelerometer steps/day translation of moderate-to-vigorous activity. Prev Med 2011;53:31–3.
13. Maceira E, Monteagudo M. Functional hallux rigidus and the Achilles-calcaneus-plantar system. Foot Ankle Clin 2014;19:669–99.

Scientific Evidence in the Treatment of Metatarsalgia

Georg Klammer, MD[a], Norman Espinosa, MD[b],*

KEYWORDS

- Metatarsalgia • Evidence • Scientific • Treatment • Review

KEY POINTS

- Metatarsalgia is a common foot disease with a multitude of causes.
- Proper identification of underlying diseases is mandatory to formulate an adequate treatment.
- Multiple surgical solutions are available to treat metatarsalgia.
- Only limited scientific evidence is available in the literature.
- However, most of the techniques used in the treatment of metatarsalgia seem to be reasonable with acceptable results.

INTRODUCTION

Metatarsalgia is a common problem in daily medical practice. The main symptom is pain, which arises underneath the second through to the fourth metatarsal heads and can be very debilitating. The clinical symptomatology varies and might be associated with the fact that the underlying causes of this kind of disease vary.

Proper diagnosis of metatarsalgia is essential to address the problem. There have been many treatment strategies formulated to improve the situation for patients. A physician can choose between nonoperative and operative strategies. But the most important question remains: Which one should be applied to provide optimal pain relief for the patient?

Physicians should always strive to ascertain the proper indication for any treatment given to a patient. However, there data are missing in this regard. Therefore, the current state of medical practice is to rely on scientific evidence, which is derived from published articles in the literature. The difficulty of distinguishing between scientifically sound and flawed articles may complicate the proper synthesis of scientific information to get a solid base for an optimal treatment.

[a] Institute for Foot and Ankle Reconstruction, Kappelistrasse 7, 8002 Zurich, Switzerland;
[b] Institute for Foot and Ankle Reconstruction, FussInsitut Zurich, Kappelistrasse 7, Zurich 8002, Switzerland
* Corresponding address.
E-mail address: espinosa@fussinsitut.ch

Foot Ankle Clin N Am 24 (2019) 585–598
https://doi.org/10.1016/j.fcl.2019.08.001
1083-7515/19/© 2019 Elsevier Inc. All rights reserved.

This article compiles all available evidence and offers a means for physicians to extract the most important information with regard to the relevant nonoperative and surgical solutions for metatarsalgia.

CLASSIFICATION

Three "rockers" have been used to define metatarsalgia. The first rocker starts at the initial contact of the heel until the foot progresses to foot flat on the ground. First rocker metatarsalgia may occur in congenital deformities, tight heel cord, or in a severe cavus foot. The second rocker starts with propulsion of the tibia over the talus and foot fall on the ground. The medial arch is maintained and at the end of this phase the triceps surae is intensively activated. Metatarsalgia occurs with limited ankle dorsiflexion or plantarflexed metatarsals. In the third rocker, the foot turns over the fixed, progressively dorsiflexed metatarsophalangeal joints and metatarsalgia occurs with deformities of these joints.[1,2]

NONOPERATIVE TREATMENT STRATEGIES

In general, nonoperative measures are initiated first to treat metatarsalgia. The single use of one of these conservative strategies, or combinations of them, may help to alleviate pain and provide reasonable effects in patients with metatarsalgia. The current paragraphs list contemporary options and evidence for their use.

Shoes and Insoles

The largest deformation of the flexible foot is found at the beginning of stance phase. During midstance it remains stable and transforms into a tight configuration at the phase of propulsion; however, no forefoot collapse occurs.[3] High plantar pressures under the metatarsal heads are associated with pain.[4] Insoles are fitted to patients with foot complaints to redistribute plantar pressures,[4–7] but designs of insoles constructed for the same patient with forefoot pain may vary significantly between experts.[8] Stolwijk and colleagues[4] examined insoles designed for variable foot complaints: the insoles showed basic similarities, but were designed significantly differently depending on whether the patient suffered from heel or forefoot pain; however, the effect on plantar pressures with a shift toward the midfoot area were similar. Various studies showed that insoles successfully redistribute pressures around the forefoot.[4–6,9]

Insoles with metatarsal support reduced peak pressures under the metatarsal heads by 11% to 22%,[5,10] likely shifting the pressure more proximal from the metatarsal heads toward the shaft.[4,6] To unload the metatarsal heads in patients with metatarsalgia tear-drop-shaped metatarsal pads often are applied. In a series of 13 patients (18 feet) suffering from metatarsalgia, Kang and colleagues found significant changes of maximal peak pressures under the 2nd metatarsal head, as well as significantly improved pain scores, after 2 weeks of treatment. Maximal peak pressures and pressure time integral before and after treatment did not improve; however, their decline did correlate to subjective pain improvement.[9]

Whereas metatarsal pads are placed on the insole, metatarsal bars are applied outside the shoe and therefore patient acceptance is worse. However, metatarsal bars show favorable results in pressure reduction compared with pads, especially when placed obliquely on the shoe instead of perpendicular.[11]

Custom-molded insoles may achieve more significant reductions of pain compared with rockerbars,[6] but in general there is no strong evidence of superiority with regard to custom-made insoles in foot complaints.[12]

Considering shoe wear, highest peak pressures were demonstrated with hard-soled shoes and lowest peak pressures were demonstrated with soft-soled shoes.[13] However, in the study by Lane and colleagues[14] with equal sole shapes no differences were observed in comfort scores in patients with forefoot pain aged over 65 years on the day of testing. Nevertheless the softer-soled shoes were preferred by most participants of the study (63%). Because a correlation has been established between pressure and pain, deterioration of metatarsalgia with wearing of hard-soled shoes over time may be supposed. However, attention must be paid to the negative influence of softer soles on stability in patients at risk of falling.

Stretching

The gastrocnemius originates with 2 separate heads from the medial and lateral femoral condyle and joins distally to the soleus muscle to build the Achilles tendon. Contraction of the gastrocnemius therefore acts on the knee joint as well as the ankle and subtalar joints. Thus, the muscle is tensioned when the knee is extended and the ankle joint in slight dorsiflexion.[15] Forefoot pressures are highest when, in this position, the tight gastrocnemius is maximally stretched.[15,16] During gait this occurs between the 60th and the 90th percentile of the stance phase.[15,17]

Restricted ankle dorsiflexion alters gait to early heel-off, subtalar overpronation, and dorsal-extension stress on the midtarsal joints and consecutive midfoot hypermobility.[18]

In patients with hallux valgus, a tight gastrocnemius can often be found,[19,20] and more than 60% of these patients also present symptoms of metatarsalgia.[20] In 66 patients with foot and ankle pain, Jastifer and Marston[21] found an ankle dorsiflexion restricted to, on average, 11.6° compared with 17.2° in the control group. Isolated gastrocnemius tightness is distinguished from tightness of the gastrocnemius-soleus complex by means of the Silfverskjöld test. It is defined positive when ankle dorsiflexion is less than 5° with the knee extended and improving to at least 10° when the knee is bent.[22]

Gastrocnemius lengthening should therefore result in decreased forefoot peak pressures and metatarsalgia.

Stretching of the myotendinous unit results in a lengthening through viscoelastic deformation.[23] The amount of deformation depends on the type and duration of stretching; however, the effect is only transient.[23] In theory, plastic or permanent deformation may occur with stretching of the tissue beyond its elastic limit; however, in practice this is not reached.[23,24] No evidence was found to support the theory that static stretch would lead to neuromuscular relaxation. If static stretching led to an increased extensibility by muscle lengthening there should be a lasting shift in the curve of passive torque and angle. However, this was not found and only end-range joint angles and applied torque increased. Thus the sensation theory was established, according to which the effect of increased myotendinous elasticity is achieved after stretching programs over 3 to 8 weeks, although the patients adapted sensation to end stretching (tension and pain). This may be a peripheral, central, or even psychological phenomenon.[23,25,26]

A successful increase of ankle dorsiflexion is reached with stretching immediately after and for up to 8 weeks.[26,27] Stretching exercises are performed with the knee extended and—if performed in a 3-week program—are equally effective under weight-bearing or non-weightbearing conditions.[28] Incorporating anteroposterior talocrural joint mobilization into the gastrocnemius stretching program will increase time to heel-off during gait and ankle dorsiflexion before heel-off.[25,29]

In summary, the evidence for the effectiveness of stretching in the treatment of metatarsalgia is limited. Nevertheless, in the case of clinically assessed contracture of the gastrocnemius it seems to be appropriate.[30] Active stretching exercises, performed 3 times daily have been advised, with a time investment averaging 20 minutes.[30] A meta-analysis including 5 studies comparing static calf muscle stretching with no stretching found a statistically significant improvement of ankle dorsiflexion of about 2° after less than 15 minutes of stretching and 3° when stretching for 15 to 30 minutes.[30,31] Efficient gait requires ankle dorsiflexion of 5° to 18°. Thus, the gain of motion reached with stretching to address metatarsalgia can be questionable.[30–32] Although studies have described a positive effect of stretching on plantar fasciitis and Achilles tendinosis,[19,33,34] we are not aware of studies examining the effect of stretching on pain or plantar pressures in patients with metatarsalgia.

Infiltration

A common cause of metatarsalgia is Morton neuroma, which is considered an entrapment neuropathy of the interdigital nerve under the transverse metatarsal ligament, and commonly attributed to mechanical overload with repetitive microtrauma.[35] Microscopic nerve degeneration with peripheral and intraneural fibrosis has been found.[36] Concomitant mechanical overload may lead to intermetatarsal bursitis, synovitis, or metatarsophalangeal joint instability.[37,38]

When Morton neuralgia becomes clinically relevant, a steroid infiltration may be considered. Earlier studies showed variable results with steroid injection,[39–41] and a Cochrane database review failed to identify relevant randomized trials.[42] However, in 2013, Thomson and colleagues[43] performed a level 1 study comparing the efficacy of ultrasound-guided intermetatarsal infiltration (1 mL 40 mg methylprednisolone and 1 mL 2% lignocaine) with a control group receiving local anesthetic infiltration alone: the steroid group showed significantly better results at global assessment of foot health, independent of neuroma size, after 3 months. Satisfaction rates of steroid infiltrations for Morton neuroma are about 45% for a single intervention, and around 75% to 80% for repeated interventions.[39–41,44] Ruiz Santiago and colleagues,[44] in a recent study, compared the satisfaction rates with blind or ultrasound-guided infiltration: satisfaction rates 15 days to 6 months postoperatively were similar to those reported earlier; however, at some stages significantly improved rates were found in the ultrasound-guided group. One should be aware that also the placebo effects show superior results with repeated treatment.[45] Earlier reports did not find improved results with ultrasound guidance, possibly because of the small sample size.[46] It has been pointed out that, in the level 1 study by Thomson and colleagues cited above, the significant positive response to the steroid injection was not maintained at 1 year.[43,47] Several other studies support this immediate to short benefit of corticoid infiltration, with the effect decreasing by 6 to 12 months.[40,41,44,47] Older patients with a short history of pain may show greater improvement from corticoid infiltration.[47]

Serious adverse events are rare; however, patients should be informed of a 5% to 10% risk of cosmetically disturbing skin hypopigmentation and fat atrophy.[43,44] Repigmentation may occur already after 1 month, but can take a year for significant recovery.[48]

In summary, steroid infiltration is a valuable treatment option to achieve pain relief in patients with Morton neuroma for at least a limited period of 3 months. We agree with other commentators that history and clinical examination in most cases is sufficient to establish the correct diagnosis and that infiltration can safely be performed without sonographic guidance.[49,50] Better satisfaction rates possibly can be achieved with sonographic guidance, but considering the costs this does not seem justified.[44]

Considering that the effect of infiltration is expected to be of short duration, patients need to be advised to the likely need for surgery in the future.[47]

Steroid infiltration in patients with metatarsalgia has been proposed in cases with metatarsophalangeal instability.[51] However, whereas steroid infiltration into the inter-metatarsal web space may help to differentiate pain between a Morton neuroma and the metatarsophalangeal joint, destabilization of the joint with deterioration of the plantar plate may be accelerated and therefore infiltration must be indicated with caution.[52]

As well as infiltration using corticosteroids, injection with alcohol-sclerosing agents, hyaloron and Botox, has been proposed.

By infiltration of Morton neuromas with mixtures of local anesthetic and ethyl alcohol (varying alcohol concentrations of 4% to 50%), favorable results were shown in the short term.[35,53-55] The minimal alcohol concentration proven to achieve neural inhibition is 20%.[56] Without use of ultrasound, success of the infiltration may be assessed by postinterventional resolution of pain. However, Espinosa and colleagues[57] were able to demonstrate that alcohol-sclerosing therapy without ultrasound guidance was not effective—possibly as a result of leakage of the solution outside the neuroma and consequent soft-tissue irritation.[54] The evidence for this treatment is limited to retrospective case series. The largest series of which was performed by Pasquali and colleagues,[54] which included 540 feet treated with injection of 50% alcohol repeated maximally 4 times until the patient was pain free. No major complication occurred and, at the 1-year follow-up, satisfaction with treatment was 75%. Gurdezi and colleagues[55] even reported 5-year results with apparent continuous success (71% satisfaction rate). Secondary neurectomy was performed in 3% to 9.3% of feet at the 10- to 12-month follow-up,[53,54] but increased to 36% at 5 years.[55] Lorenzon and Rettore[35] associated failures of alcohol-sclerosing therapy to unaddressed mechanical metatarsalgia, because alcohol injection does not lead to necrosis or apoptosis and some axonal regrowth occurs, and mechanical overload persists if unaddressed.[35] Being aware of the probable mechanical cause of Morton neuroma, one should always consider addressing the causes of mechanical overload, and possible concomitant synovitis and metatarsophalangeal instability, respectively. This is more common when the 2nd to 3rd intermetatarsal webspace is affected, and therefore should influence our conservative or surgical treatment plan.[35,37]

Radiofrequency Ablation of Morton Neuroma

Another proposed treatment modality for Morton neuroma to avoid surgical complications is radiofrequency ablation. Evidence is limited to few case series.[58,59] Chuter and colleagues[59] included 30 feet in 25 patients: after an average of 1.6 treatments with ultrasound guidance and a minimum follow-up of 6 months, satisfactory outcome was reported in 87%, with a 10% progression to surgical excision. However, with lack of a control group the results could be biased by the concomitant infiltration of steroids to reduce postprocedural pain. In a study by Brooks and colleagues,[60] 3 cycles of radiofrequency ablation seemed superior to 2 cycles, with satisfaction rates of 88% and 12.5%, with secondary neurectomy after a follow-up of an average of 13 months. As with the injection of sclerosing ethyl agents, sonographically guided treatment seems favorable.[58-60] Complications range from temporary nerve irritation to metatarsal bone necrosis.[59] The intervention needs to be performed in the operating theater under local anesthetic block, analgosedation, or even general anesthesia. Considering the costs, better evidence is required to justify more widespread application of the technique.

SURGICAL TREATMENT STRATEGIES
Gastrocnemius Release

The indication for a surgical gastrocnemius release is a failed conservative treatment regarding muscle stretching. However, the final goal is the same in the latter and focuses on reduction of pressure at the forefoot. There are 5 distinct levels where a gastrocnemius release could be performed. Silfverskjöld proposed a proximal release, which has been modified to the proximal medial gastrocnemius release.[30,31] In contrast to Silfverskjöld, Baumann suggested a proximal but deep gastrocnemius release, which is a little bit more demanding from a surgeon's perspective.[61] Instead of performing a proximal release, Strayer[62] proposed a release closer to the musculotendinous unit. This technique is quite similar to that suggested by Vulpius and Stoffel[63] and Baker.[64] All of these techniques require 1 specific underlying condition: a short or contracted gastrocnemius complex, which results in a positive Silfverskjöld test. In the presence of a negative Silfverskjöld test but contracted calf musculature, the sole release of the gastrocnemius would not be effective. In those cases, the Achilles tendon needs to be lengthened, which can be done as previously described.[65–67]

A recent paper published by Morales-Muñoz and colleagues[68] (level IV, case series) showed an improvement of ankle dorsiflexion and reduction of visual-analog scales in patients with metatarsalgia. All patients underwent a proximal medial gastrocnemius release. The effect on function and strength after gastrocnemius recession were acceptable, including increased range of motion while not affecting strength in plantarflexion.[69,70] Similar results have been found for the Strayer procedure.[71]

Endoscopically performed releases have become a new way to improve cosmetics and morbidity in patients with gastrocnemius contracture. Phisitkul and colleagues[32] presented the results from their prospective study (level IV, case series) in 320 consecutive patients, and were able to confirm a high level of surgical safety as well as improved ankle dorsiflexion and improvement of pain after resection.

Cychosz and colleagues[18] reviewed the literature (level IV, systematic review) to investigate the evidence for gastrocnemius recession for foot and ankle pathologies, and found only a grade B evidence ("fair") to support the use of gastrocnemius recession for the treatment of isolated foot pain owing to midfoot/forefoot overload syndrome in adults. As well as this, the authors were able to identify certain data supporting the use of gastrocnemius recession to treat midfoot or forefoot ulcers and noninsertional Achilles tendinopathy in adults, but to date this evidence remains grade C.

First Ray Hypermobility and Its Treatment

The medial column of the foot absorbs almost 60% of weight during normal weight-bearing from the heel strike to toe-off. However, in case of first ray insufficiency as—for example—seen in hallux valgus deformity, the load might become shifted laterally to the lesser metatarsal and create overload, which in turn results in metatarsalgia. Whether the hypermobility of the first ray is the cause of hallux valgus deformity in some feet, and if it should be treated, is currently debated. The concept of an increased mobility of the first ray was firstly introduced by Morton,[72] and first clinically assessed by Couarriades[73] as an increased mobility in extension of the first tarsometatarsal joint when the lesser metatarsal heads were held in the hand. During recent years the existence of hypermobility of the first ray has been questioned, although it has been confirmed and measured in cadavers.[74,75]

The question concerning the possible relationship of hypermobility of the first ray with hallux valgus deformity needs to be addressed. To answer this question, Klaue and colleagues[76] created a device to assess the hypermobility of the first ray in feet with hallux valgus deformity and compared the measurements with those in feet without deformity. They concluded that the first metatarsal can shift dorsally up 8 mm while being considered normal.[76] In addition, there is evidence of statically significant mean differences between feet with deformity and those without of 3.62 mm (95% confidence interval 2.26–4.98).[38,77] This difference can differ from the position of the ankle[77]: in plantarflexion the mobility becomes greater than in dorsiflexion of the ankle. The test should be performed with the ankle in a neutral position, but the authors do not agree with this. They suggest performing the test during maximum dorsiflexion of the ankle. In this way, the flexors become fully tensioned and should prevent any hyperflexion or hyperextension. Therefore, from a clinical point of view, the authors classify hypermobility of the first ray as either present or absent—nothing else.

Greisberg and colleagues[78] described an evident correlation between first ray hypermobility and preoperative hallux valgus angle ($r = 0.178$ $P = .052$), as well as an increased 1st to 2nd intermetatarsal angle ($r = 0.181$ $P = .048$). This suggests that the sagittal motion of the first cuneio-metatarsal joint might be one of the causes of many cases of hallux valgus and, consequently, also a cause of metatarsalgia. Greisberg and colleagues[79] also demonstrated that those patients with metatarsalgia and hallux valgus had a greater significantly first ray mobility and mean metatarsal elevation. In contrast, feet with low arches have shown greater mobility than those with high arches, and patients with hallux rigidus showed decreased mobility.[80]

In conclusion, first ray mobility on average is increased in patients with hallux valgus and is increased in some patients with transfer metatarsalgia.

Distal Metatarsal Osteotomies

Since its first description in 1985 by Weil, this type of osteotomy has become an important surgical means of treating central, third-rocker metatarsalgia. In recent years, several surgical modifications have been introduced to reduce the potential complications associated with this kind of operative intervention but most of them have not proven to be better than the original one.

The concept of the Weil osteotomy consists of metatarsal shortening. However, the center of rotation can become plantarflexed, altering the biomechanics of the metatarsophalangeal joints and leading to dorsiflexion of the toes, an entity called "floating-toe" deformity. In an attempt to avoid this kind of complication, the Weil osteotomy has been modified by resecting a bone block or wedge from the osteotomy site. Nevertheless, even this particular modification did not prove to have any advantage over the original procedure.

The current literature reveals good-to-excellent results in 70% to 100% of patients who have been treated by means of conventional Weil osteotomy.[81–83] However, stiffness at the metatarsophalangeal joints and floating-toe deformities still remain.[81] The authors believe that most of the stiff and floating-toes might be associated with postoperative scar tissue. In addition, the classic Weil osteotomy and its modifications are all intraarticular osteotomies requiring an open approach.

To prevent these complications and to allow better outcomes, percutaneous techniques have been introduced. In contrast to the open techniques, percutaneous surgeries act extra-articularly and may avoid scarring of the joint capsule, which could be seen as a potential factor for postoperative joint stiffness. When performing a percutaneous distal metatarsal metaphyseal osteotomy (DMMO), the position of the head fragment is dictated by the soft-tissue tension and pressure exerted during weight bearing. In addition, shortening and slight elevation can be achieved. However, the lack of fixation itself could be a risk factor for nonunion, which in turn may be very difficult to treat.

Most published articles regarding distal metatarsal osteotomies focus on open techniques and lack proper scientific evidence (level IV).

In 2011, Besse and Fessy[82] published a level III, comparative and retrospective study comparing the Weil osteotomy with the percutaneous DMMO technique. Interestingly, the results were similar in both groups at final follow-up (14 months) with no superior results in the percutaneous DMMO group considering range of motion. A greater portion of patients in the percutaneous DMMO group showed normal mobility (or slight impairment), but this was not statistically significant. On the other hand, edema was more frequently found in the percutaneous group, resulting in prolonged recovery after surgery.

Similar results were found in 2018 by Johansen and colleagues[83] (level II, prospective, comparative and randomized study). The differences between the groups in this prospective and randomized study were small, with no possibility to draw any conclusion in favor of the percutaneous DMMO technique. Importantly, tourniquet time and operating time were lower in the percutaneous DMMO group, but radiation doses were higher compared with the open Weil osteotomies.

Finally, there is no sound scientific evidence regarding the effects of either open or percutaneous techniques in the treatment of metatarsalgia. However, most published papers report a positive tendency in terms of pressure relief and adequate functional results. Future studies are needed to improve the understanding of distal metatarsal osteotomies.

Metatarsal Shaft Osteotomies

In 1954, Giannestras[84] was first to describe a step-cut osteotomy for the treatment of plantar keratoses. However, instead of elevating, the procedure shortened the metatarsal bone. In contrast, midshaft segmental osteotomy (as described by Hansen[85]) allows coaxial shortening of an elevation of the metatarsal bone and head, respectively. Spence and colleagues[86] reported on this technique without internal fixation and revealed good-to-excellent results in 89% of patients. Although many patients were satisfied with the procedure, radiographic evidence of nonunion was seen in 76%, which is far too high to recommend such an intervention. To avoid nonunions, Galluch and colleagues[87] modified the technique by application of a dorsally placed and prebent plate. Prebending the plate offers plantar compression and secures the osteotomy site by creation of even pressure distributions. As confirmed by a retrospective (level IV) study, the union rate was found to average 99.2% after a follow-up interval of 5 to 18 months. The patient population (N = 95) in this study was not homogenous, and therefore the results must be interpreted with caution. In 2015, DeSandis and colleagues[88] published their results (level IV) of midshaft segmental shortening procedures in 58 patients (91 osteotomies). The same problem as seen in the study by Galluch and colleagues[87] was also seen in this study. The inhomogenous patient population, with many additional surgeries, did not allow to draw sound conclusions on this kind of treatment. The nonunion rate at 6 months postoperatively was still quite high (22 osteotomies), but improved until 13 months postoperatively (93%). Thus, union of the metatarsals in those patients needs to be considered over a long period of time.

To conclude, it must be said that there is no high-class scientific evidence to support this kind of treatment for metatarsalgia, but most of the published literature dealing with this topic reveals acceptable and good results.

PROXIMAL METATARSAL OSTEOTOMIES

The proper indication for any proximal metatarsal osteotomy is a patient suffering from second-rocker metatarsalgia.

Proximal osteotomies of the central metatarsals were first mentioned by Khoury Sola and colleagues[89] in 1970, and were then further developed by Aiello[90] in 1981. Aiello reported on either a single or double V-shaped proximal metaphyseal bone osteotomy. As reported by Aiello, 89% of patients were satisfied with the treatment (85 feet in 45 patients). Harper[91] presented his experience with proximal dorsal closed-wedge osteotomies and provided a trigonometric analysis. Harper's paper focused on the great power of correction and the relation between the size of the wedge and elevation and/or shortening of metatarsal bones. More recently, Barouk and colleagues[92] reported the so-called Barouk-Rippstein-Toullec osteotomy to treat second-rocker metatarsalgia. However, the concept is almost identical to that of Harper, who commented on this in 1990.[91] In 2014, Gougoulias and Sakellariou[93] reported on the results of a proximal closing wedge osteotomy to correct medial or lateral subluxation of the lesser toes. However, the study included only 4 patients. All patients maintained clinical and radiographic outcome after 12 months of follow-up.

Proximal osteotomies are powerful means to correct metatarsalgia of second-rocker type but are technically challenging procedures. Although some studies exist in the literature, the scientific evidence is weak and therefore further studies are needed to confirm its true effectiveness in patients with metatarsalgia.

SUMMARY

In summary, there is not much scientific evidence for any conservative or surgical treatment in cases of metatarsalgia. Scientific evidence at a high level requires large patient populations and very sound study designs. However, many articles are available and demonstrate adequate results, which in turn may help physicians to treat metatarsalgia in a satisfactory way. When looking at more recent publications, the data offer a solid base to decide on which kind of treatment a physician should embark on or not. The authors hope that in future better evidence can be elaborated. Nevertheless, most of the techniques and approaches mentioned in this article have become reliable and satisfying treatment strategies. These techniques are the basis for future scientific research.

ACKNOWLEDGMENTS

The authors would like to thank Laia Lopez Capdevila, MD, for her contributions to this article.

REFERENCES

1. Mayich DJ, Novak A, Vena D, et al. Gait analysis in orthopedic foot and ankle surgery—topical review, part 1: principles and uses of gait analysis. Foot Ankle Int 2014;35(1):80–90.
2. Espinosa N, Brodsky JW, Maceira E. Metatarsalgia. J Am Acad Orthop Surg 2010;18(8):474–85.
3. Duerinck S, Hagman F, Jonkers I, et al. Forefoot deformation during stance: does the forefoot collapse during loading? Gait Posture 2014;39(1):40–7.
4. Stolwijk NM, Louwerens JWK, Nienhuis B, et al. Plantar pressure with and without custom insoles in patients with common foot complaints. Foot Ankle Int 2011; 32(1):57–65.

5. Hodge MC, Bach TM, Carter GM. Novel Award First Prize Paper. Orthotic management of plantar pressure and pain in rheumatoid arthritis. Clin Biomech (Bristol Avon) 1999;14(8):567–75.

6. Postema K, Burm PE, Zande ME, et al. Primary metatarsalgia: the influence of a custom moulded insole and a rockerbar on plantar pressure. Prosthet Orthot Int 1998;22(1):35–44.

7. Tsung BYS, Zhang M, Mak AFT, et al. Effectiveness of insoles on plantar pressure redistribution. J Rehabil Res Dev 2004;41(6A):767–74.

8. Guldemond NA, Leffers P, Schaper NC, et al. Comparison of foot orthoses made by podiatrists, pedorthists and orthotists regarding plantar pressure reduction in the Netherlands. BMC Musculoskelet Disord 2005;6:61.

9. Kang J-H, Chen M-D, Chen S-C, et al. Correlations between subjective treatment responses and plantar pressure parameters of metatarsal pad treatment in metatarsalgia patients: a prospective study. BMC Musculoskelet Disord 2006;7:95.

10. Chang B-C, Liu D-H, Chang JL, et al. Plantar pressure analysis of accommodative insole in older people with metatarsalgia. Gait Posture 2014;39(1):449–54.

11. Deshaies A, Roy P, Symeonidis PD, et al. Metatarsal bars more effective than metatarsal pads in reducing impulse on the second metatarsal head. Foot (Edinb) 2011;21(4):172–5.

12. Nawoczenski DA, Janisse DJ. Foot orthoses in rehabilitation—what's new. Clin Sports Med 2004;23(1):157–67.

13. Jarboe NE, Quesada PM. The effects of cycling shoe stiffness on forefoot pressure. Foot Ankle Int 2003;24(10):784–8.

14. Lane TJ, Landorf KB, Bonanno DR, et al. Effects of shoe sole hardness on plantar pressure and comfort in older people with forefoot pain. Gait Posture 2014;39(1):247–51.

15. Cazeau C, Stiglitz Y. Effects of gastrocnemius tightness on forefoot during gait. Foot Ankle Clin 2014;19(4):649–57.

16. Aronow MS, Diaz-Doran V, Sullivan RJ, et al. The effect of triceps surae contracture force on plantar foot pressure distribution. Foot Ankle Int 2006;27(1):43–52.

17. Espinosa N, Maceira E, Myerson MS. Current concept review: metatarsalgia. Foot Ankle Int 2008;29(8):871–9.

18. Cychosz CC, Phisitkul P, Belatti DA, et al. Gastrocnemius recession for foot and ankle conditions in adults: evidence-based recommendations. Foot Ankle Surg 2015;21(2):77–85.

19. DiGiovanni CW, Kuo R, Tejwani N, et al. Isolated gastrocnemius tightness. J Bone Joint Surg Am 2002;84-A(6):962–70.

20. Barouk P. Recurrent metatarsalgia. Foot Ankle Clin 2014;19(3):407–24.

21. Jastifer JR, Marston J. Gastrocnemius contracture in patients with and without foot pathology. Foot Ankle Int 2016;37(11):1165–70.

22. Silfverskiold N. Reduction of the uncrossed two joints muscles of the leg to one joint muscles in spastic conditions. Acta Chir Scand 1924;(56):315–30.

23. Weppler CH, Magnusson SP. Increasing muscle extensibility: a matter of increasing length or modifying sensation? Phys Ther 2010;90(3):438–49.

24. Feland JB, Myrer JW, Schulthies SS, et al. The effect of duration of stretching of the hamstring muscle group for increasing range of motion in people aged 65 years or older. Phys Ther 2001;81(5):1110–7.

25. Kang M-H, Oh J-S, Kwon O-Y, et al. Immediate combined effect of gastrocnemius stretching and sustained talocrural joint mobilization in individuals with limited ankle dorsiflexion: a randomized controlled trial. Man Ther 2015;20(6):827–34.

26. Halbertsma JP, Göeken LN. Stretching exercises: effect on passive extensibility and stiffness in short hamstrings of healthy subjects. Arch Phys Med Rehabil 1994;75(9):976–81.
27. Magnusson SP, Aagard P, Simonsen E, et al. A biomechanical evaluation of cyclic and static stretch in human skeletal muscle. Int J Sports Med 1998;19(5):310–6.
28. Dinh NV, Freeman H, Granger J, et al. Calf stretching in non-weight bearing versus weight bearing. Int J Sports Med 2011;32(3):205–10.
29. Kang M-H, Lee D-K, Kim S-Y, et al. The influence of gastrocnemius stretching combined with joint mobilization on weight-bearing ankle dorsiflexion passive range of motion. J Phys Ther Sci 2015;27(5):1317–8.
30. Cortina RE, Morris BL, Vopat BG. Gastrocnemius recession for metatarsalgia. Foot Ankle Clin 2018;23(1):57–68.
31. Radford JA, Burns J, Buchbinder R, et al. Does stretching increase ankle dorsiflexion range of motion? A systematic review. Br J Sports Med 2006;40(10):870–5 [discussion: 875].
32. Phisitkul P, Rungprai C, Femino JE, et al. Endoscopic gastrocnemius recession for the treatment of isolated gastrocnemius contracture: a prospective study on 320 consecutive patients. Foot Ankle Int 2014;35(8):747–56.
33. Courville XF, Coe MP, Hecht PJ. Current concepts review: noninsertional Achilles tendinopathy. Foot Ankle Int 2009;30(11):1132–42.
34. Barske HL, DiGiovanni BF, Douglass M, et al. Current concepts review: isolated gastrocnemius contracture and gastrocnemius recession. Foot Ankle Int 2012; 33(10):915–21.
35. Lorenzon P, Rettore C. Mechanical metatarsalgia as a risk factor for relapse of Morton's neuroma after ultrasound-guided alcohol injection. J Foot Ankle Surg 2018;57(5):870–5.
36. Giannini S, Bacchini P, Ceccarelli F, et al. Interdigital neuroma: clinical examination and histopathologic results in 63 cases treated with excision. Foot Ankle Int 2004;25(2):79–84.
37. Bauer T, Golano P, Hardy P. Endoscopic resection of a calcaneonavicular coalition. Knee Surg Sports Traumatol Arthrosc 2010;18(5):669–72.
38. Coughlin MJ, Schenck RC, Shurnas PS, et al. Concurrent interdigital neuroma and MTP joint instability: long-term results of treatment. Foot Ankle Int 2002; 23(11):1018–25.
39. Bennett GL, Graham CE, Mauldin DM. Morton's interdigital neuroma: a comprehensive treatment protocol. Foot Ankle Int 1995;16(12):760–3.
40. Rasmussen MR, Kitaoka HB, Patzer GL. Nonoperative treatment of plantar interdigital neuroma with a single corticosteroid injection. Clin Orthop 1996;326: 188–93.
41. Saygi B, Yildirim Y, Saygi EK, et al. Morton neuroma: comparative results of two conservative methods. Foot Ankle Int 2005;26(7):556–9.
42. Thomson CE, Gibson JNA, Martin D. Interventions for the treatment of Morton's neuroma. Cochrane Database Syst Rev 2004;(3):CD003118.
43. Thomson CE, Beggs I, Martin DJ, et al. Methylprednisolone injections for the treatment of Morton neuroma: a patient-blinded randomized trial. J Bone Joint Surg Am 2013;95(9):790–8. S1.
44. Ruiz Santiago F, Prados Olleta N, Tomás Muñoz P, et al. Short term comparison between blind and ultrasound guided injection in Morton neuroma. Eur Radiol 2018. https://doi.org/10.1007/s00330-018-5670-1.
45. Hróbjartsson A, Gøtzsche PC. Placebo interventions for all clinical conditions. Cochrane Database Syst Rev 2010;(1):CD003974.

46. Mahadevan D, Venkatesan M, Bhatt R, et al. Diagnostic accuracy of clinical tests for Morton's neuroma compared with ultrasonography. J Foot Ankle Surg 2015; 54(4):549–53.
47. Lizano-Díez X, Ginés-Cespedosa A, Alentorn-Geli E, et al. Corticosteroid injection for the treatment of Morton's neuroma: a prospective, double-blinded, randomized, placebo-controlled trial. Foot Ankle Int 2017;38(9):944–51.
48. van Vendeloo SN, Ettema HB. Skin depigmentation along lymph vessels of the lower leg following local corticosteroid injection for interdigital neuroma. Foot Ankle Surg 2016;22(2):139–41.
49. Schon L. An injection of corticosteroid plus anesthetic was more effective than anesthetic alone for Morton neuroma. J Bone Joint Surg Am 2014;96(4):334.
50. Smith RW. Steroid injection for Morton neuroma—data-based justification. J Bone Joint Surg Am 2013;95(9):e64.
51. Trepman E, Yeo SJ. Nonoperative treatment of metatarsophalangeal joint synovitis. Foot Ankle Int 1995;16(12):771–7.
52. DiPreta JA. Metatarsalgia, lesser toe deformities, and associated disorders of the forefoot. Med Clin North Am 2014;98(2):233–51.
53. Hughes RJ, Ali K, Jones H, et al. Treatment of Morton's neuroma with alcohol injection under sonographic guidance: follow-up of 101 cases. AJR Am J Roentgenol 2007;188(6):1535–9.
54. Pasquali C, Vulcano E, Novario R, et al. Ultrasound-guided alcohol injection for Morton's neuroma. Foot Ankle Int 2015;36(1):55–9.
55. Gurdezi S, White T, Ramesh P. Alcohol injection for Morton's neuroma: a five-year follow-up. Foot Ankle Int 2013;34(8):1064–7.
56. Rengachary SS, Watanabe IS, Singer P, et al. Effect of glycerol on peripheral nerve: an experimental study. Neurosurgery 1983;13(6):681–8.
57. Espinosa N, Seybold JD, Jankauskas L, et al. Alcohol sclerosing therapy is not an effective treatment for interdigital neuroma. Foot Ankle Int 2011;32(6):576–80.
58. Genon MP, Chin TY, Bedi HS, et al. Radio-frequency ablation for the treatment of Morton's neuroma. ANZ J Surg 2010;80(9):583–5.
59. Chuter GSJ, Chua YP, Connell DA, et al. Ultrasound-guided radiofrequency ablation in the management of interdigital (Morton's) neuroma. Skeletal Radiol 2013; 42(1):107–11.
60. Brooks D, Parr A, Bryceson W. Three cycles of radiofrequency ablation are more efficacious than two in the management of Morton's neuroma. Foot Ankle Spec 2018;11(2):107–11.
61. Baumann JU. Ventrale aponeurotische Verlängerung des Musculus gastrocnemius. Oper Orthop Traumatol 1989;(1):254–8.
62. Strayer LM. Recession of the gastrocnemius; an operation to relieve spastic contracture of the calf muscles. J Bone Joint Surg Am 1950;32-A(3):671–6.
63. Vulpius OS, Stoffel A. Orthopädische Operationslehre: Tenotomie der Endsehnen der Mm Gastrocnemius et Soleus mittels Rutschenlassens nach Vulpius. Stuttgart (Germany): Ferdinand Enke; 1913. p. 29–31.
64. Baker LD. A rational approach to the surgical needs of the cerebral palsy patient. J Bone Joint Surg Am 1956;38-A(2):313–23.
65. Hoke M. An operation for the correction of extremely relaxed flat feet. J Bone Joint Surg 1931;(13):773–83.
66. White JW. Torsion of the Achilles tendon: its surgical significance. Arch Surg 1943;46:784–7.
67. Herzenberg JE, Lamm BM, Corwin C, et al. Isolated recession of the gastrocnemius muscle: the Baumann procedure. Foot Ankle Int 2007;28(11):1154–9.

68. Morales-Muñoz P, De Los Santos Real R, Barrio Sanz P, et al. Proximal gastrocnemius release in the treatment of mechanical metatarsalgia. Foot Ankle Int 2016;37(7):782–9.
69. Chimera NJ, Castro M, Manal K. Function and strength following gastrocnemius recession for isolated gastrocnemius contracture. Foot Ankle Int 2010;31(5): 377–84.
70. Maskill JD, Bohay DR, Anderson JG. Gastrocnemius recession to treat isolated foot pain. Foot Ankle Int 2010;31(1):19–23.
71. Holtmann JA, Südkamp NP, Schmal H, et al. Gastrocnemius recession leads to increased ankle motion and improved patient satisfaction after 2 years of follow-up. J Foot Ankle Surg 2017;56(3):589–93.
72. Morton DJ. Hallux valgus, allied deformities of the forefoot and metatarsalgia. Chicago: Saunders Ed; 1965. p. 368–72.
73. Courriades H. L'hypermobilité du 1er rayon. Podologie 1971;6:146.
74. Wanivenhaus A, Pretterklieber M. First tarsometatarsal joint: anatomical biomechanical study. Foot Ankle 1989;9(4):153–7.
75. Gellman H, Lenihan M, Halikis N, et al. Selective tarsal arthrodesis: an in vitro analysis of the effect on foot motion. Foot Ankle 1987;8(3):127–33.
76. Klaue K, Hansen ST, Masquelet AC. Clinical, quantitative assessment of first tarsometatarsal mobility in the sagittal plane and its relation to hallux valgus deformity. Foot Ankle Int 1994;15(1):9–13.
77. Singh D, Biz C, Corradin M, et al. Comparison of dorsal and dorsomedial displacement in evaluation of first ray hypermobility in feet with and without hallux valgus. Foot Ankle Surg 2016;22(2):120–4.
78. Greisberg J, Prince D, Sperber L. First ray mobility increase in patients with metatarsalgia. Foot Ankle Int 2010;31(11):954–8.
79. Greisberg J, Sperber L, Prince DE. Mobility of the first ray in various foot disorders. Foot Ankle Int 2012;33(1):44–9.
80. Grebing BR, Coughlin MJ. The effect of ankle position on the exam for first ray mobility. Foot Ankle Int 2004;25(7):467–75.
81. Migues A, Slullitel G, Bilbao F, et al. Floating-toe deformity as a complication of the Weil osteotomy. Foot Ankle Int 2004;25(9):609–13.
82. Henry J, Besse JL, Fessy MH, et al. Distal osteotomy of the lateral metatarsals: a series of 72 cases comparing the Weil osteotomy and the DMMO percutaneous osteotomy. Orthop Traumatol Surg Res 2011;97(6 Suppl):S57–65.
83. Johansen JK, Jordan M, Thomas M. Clinical and radiological outcomes after Weil osteotomy compared to distal metatarsal metaphyseal osteotomy in the treatment of metatarsalgia—a prospective study. Foot Ankle Surg 2018. https://doi.org/10.1016/j.fas.2018.03.002.
84. Giannestras NJ. Shortening of the metatarsal shaft in the treatment of plantar keratosis; an end-result study. J Bone Joint Surg Am 1958;40-A(1):61–71.
85. Hansen ST. Functional reconstruction of the foot and ankle. Philadelphia: Lippincott Williams & Wilkins; 2000.
86. Spence KF, O'Connell SJ, Kenzora JE. Proximal metatarsal segmental resection: a treatment for intractable plantar keratoses. Orthopedics 1990;13(7):741–7.
87. Galluch DB, Bohay DR, Anderson JG. Midshaft metatarsal segmental osteotomy with open reduction and internal fixation. Foot Ankle Int 2007;28(2):169–74.
88. DeSandis B, Ellis SJ, Levitsky M, et al. Rate of union after segmental midshaft shortening osteotomy of the lesser metatarsals. Foot Ankle Int 2015;36(10): 1190–5.

89. Khoury Sola C, Llorente CA, Lardone JM. Metatarsalgia caused by mechanical changes of the anterior arch. Proximal osteotomy of the central metatarsals. Prensa Med Argent 1970;57:1825.
90. Aiello CL. Surgical treatment of metatarsalgia. Int Orthop 1981;5(2):107–9.
91. Harper MC. Dorsal closing wedge metatarsal osteotomy: a trigonometric analysis. Foot Ankle 1990;10(6):303–5.
92. Barouk LS, Barouk P. Hallux valgus et gastrocnemiens courts: etude de deux series cliniques. Brievete des gastrocnémiens. Montpellier (France): Sauramps; 2012.
93. Gougoulias N, Sakellariou A. Proximal closing wedge lesser metatarsal osteotomy for metatarsophalangeal joint transverse plane realignment. Surgical technique and outcome. Foot Ankle Surg 2014;20(1):30–3.

Evolution of the Weil Osteotomy: The Triple Osteotomy

Manuel Monteagudo, MD[a],*, Ernesto Maceira, MD[b]

KEYWORDS

- Metatarsal • Metatarsalgia • Metatarsal osteotomy • Weil • Triple-cut weil
- Floating toe

KEY POINTS

- Weil osteotomy (WO) is the most common technique worldwide for the treatment of mechanical metatarsalgia. It was developed by Lowell Weil (Chicago, US) and popularized in Europe by Samuel Barouk (Bordeaux, France).
- The main indication for WO is propulsive/third rocker metatarsalgia that is in relation with an abnormal length of a certain metatarsal with respect to the neighboring metatarsals in the frontal plane.
- Meticulous knowledge of surgical anatomy of the lesser metatarsals and surgical technique is important to avoid complications associated with WO.
- Most clinical studies have showed good to excellent results after WO. However, complications such as floating toes led to the evolution of WO and the development of the triple-cut WO.
- Ernesto Maceira (Madrid, Spain) designed and popularized triple-cut modification of WO that allows for shortening coaxial to the shaft without plantar translation of metatarsal head. Other variations of WO allow for the treatment of crossover/overriding toes, metatarsophalangeal dislocations, and second space syndrome.

 Video content accompanies this article at http://www.foot.theclinics.com.

INTRODUCTION: HISTORY OF WEIL OSTEOTOMY

Surgical treatment of metatarsalgia has been a controversial issue for decades. Some 20 years ago, no clear definition of the different types of metatarsalgia led to perform the same procedure for any type of forefoot plantar pain. More than 25 different

Disclosure Statement: The authors have no professional or financial affiliations for themselves or their spouses.
[a] Orthopaedic Foot and Ankle Unit, Orthopaedic and Trauma Department, Hospital Universitario Quirónsalud Madrid, Faculty Medicine UEM Madrid, Madrid, Spain; [b] Orthopaedica Foot and Ankle Unit, Complejo Hospitalario La Mancha Centro, Av de la Constitución 3, 13600, Alcázar de San Juan, Ciudad Real, Spain
* Corresponding author. Manuel Monteagudo Hospital, Universitario Quirónsalud Madrid, Calle Diego de Velázquez 1, Pozuelo de Alarcón, Madrid 28223, Spain.
E-mail address: mmontyr@yahoo.com

osteotomies have been described with techniques such as distal shortening osteotomies, diaphyseal shortening osteotomies, distal dorsiflexory osteotomies, proximal dorsiflexory osteotomies, condylectomies, and partial or complete metatarsal head resections.[1] It is no wonder lesser metatarsal surgery had been historically associated with poor results in the second half of the twentieth century. Many of those osteotomies were incorrectly indicated, unstable, without fixation, and with early weight bearing, thus resulting in unpredictable shortening-elevation-malunion.

In the 1990s, a better understanding of forefoot biomechanics led to the differentiation between metatarsalgia generated within the second rocker of gait and metatarsalgia generated within the third rocker of gait.[2] The rocker theory by Perry provided a simple but complete theoretic and practical framework for the understanding of the causes of metatarsalgia.[3] It was then evident that not until the cause of metatarsalgia was identified could the surgeon consider which osteotomy was suitable for the patient.

Second rocker metatarsalgia is developed because of an abnormal gastrocnemius tightness and/or abnormal attack/declination angle of a metatarsal in the sagittal plane. Surgical treatment should consider gastrocnemius lengthening and/or dorsiflexory metatarsal osteotomies to relieve plantar pressure.[3,4] *Third rocker metatarsalgia* depends on the relative length among the lesser metatarsals and with respect to the first metatarsal at toe-off. It responds well to shortening osteotomies that restore a harmonic metatarsal parabola in the frontal plane (without disturbing alignment in the sagittal plane).[4]

But in the 1980s, the problem was most osteotomies shortened metatarsals at the expense of elevation, so results were largely unpredictable. Lowell Scott Weil, a podiatrist from Chicago, designed a distal metatarsal osteotomy made parallel to the weight-bearing surface that provided axial decompression by sliding the metatarsal head proximally. Weil osteotomy (WO) was first performed in a real patient by L.S. Weil in Chicago in 1985. Louis Samuel Barouk, a French orthopedic surgeon based in Bordeaux, met Lowell Weil at a congress in Chicago in 1991. They shared experiences on forefoot reconstruction, especially the scarf osteotomy and lesser metatarsal osteotomies. In 1992, Weil was invited by Barouk to a meeting in Bordeaux on the scarf osteotomy. It was in a live surgery case at that meeting that Weil performed his metatarsal osteotomy for the first time in Europe. Barouk adopted this technique with passion and popularized WO among European orthopedic surgeons for years to come.[5] By then, it was known that most metatarsalgia cases were associated to abnormal length relationships between neighboring metatarsals (third rocker metatarsalgia). WO provided an accurate, controlled, and precise shortening of a lesser metatarsal as no other osteotomy to date.

The first formal paper on WO was published by Barouk in the German journal Orthopade in 1996.[6] Since 1990, Barouk ran training courses on forefoot reconstruction in Bordeaux showing how to plan and perform metatarsals osteotomies, including WO. Hundreds of orthopedic surgeons adopted WO as their osteotomy of choice when performing forefoot surgery. In 2003, the book Forefoot Reconstruction by LS Barouk made WO even more popular through many practical cases and WO became the most popular metatarsal osteotomy worldwide.[5]

WO gained in popularity based on the simple surgical technique, stable fixation, excellent union rates, low complication rates, and predictable results, in a time when the alternatives of Helal or diaphyseal osteotomies frequently led to uncontrolled shortening and/or elevation of a metatarsal. However, complications associated to WO existed and continue to exist to our days. Floating toes were favored by a plantar flexion displacement of the metatarsal head that occurred with shortenings greater than 3 mm. The triple(-cut) WO was later designed by Ernesto Maceira (senior author) to produce controlled shortening coaxial to the metatarsal shaft and elevation of the head that compensated for the plantar displacement generated with shortenings greater than 3 mm.[7,8]

This paper focuses on WO and tries to provide a basic understanding of the indications, technique, complications, pathomechanics, and variations. It will fundamentally address the evolution from the simple Weil to the triple(-cut) WO.

CONCEPT AND INDICATIONS

WO is a cervicocephalic controlled shortening, proximal sliding, and lesser metatarsal osteotomy that allows for the realignment of the relative lengths of the metatarsals to achieve an ideal anatomic metatarsal parabola.

In order to understand the pathomechanics of metatarsalgia and the indication of WO, the authors will refer to the "rockers" from gait analysis.[3] The contact pattern between the foot and the ground varies during the stance phase. During the second rocker of gait, abnormal metatarsal declination angle, either anatomic (pes cavus, plantarflexed metatarsals) or functional (equinism), is the key factor to understand the development of *nonpropulsive/second rocker metatarsalgia*. Metatarsal length is not relevant during static stance or during midstance, while the foot is plantigrade on the ground. Mechanical impairments that may overload the forefoot during plantigrade support are not an indication for a conventional WO.[8] Performing a WO in a patient with second rocker metatarsalgia would only displace pain and keratosis proximally and would potentially worsen the condition because of the associated lowering of the metatarsal head. However, variations of WO, such as dorsiflexory or double-cut osteotomies, might be of help in the management of second rocker metatarsalgia.

During the third rocker of gait, metatarsal length is a major etiopathogenic factor in the generation of *propulsive/third rocker metatarsalgia*. The ideal metatarsal parabola is that which allows for an even distribution of axial loading on all of the metatarsal heads during propulsion, without the need for participation of active elements.[8,9] All of the metatarsal radiographic formulas are normal as long as the foot is painless and functional. Disease takes place when the foot turns into being symptomatic. The presence of a third rocker keratosis and pain can be due to the excessive length of the corresponding metatarsal with respect to the neighboring metatarsals or the shortening of an adjacent metatarsal (**Fig. 1**). WO and shortening variations (triple-cut WO) are indicated for patients who suffer from third rocker metatarsalgia.

In cases where nonoperative treatments have failed, third rocker/propulsive metatarsalgia may benefit from osteotomies that restore the relative length among the lesser metatarsals to recreate a harmonic metatarsal parabola. WO has replaced many of the preceeding osteotomies due to its capacity to shorten the metatarsal without significant elevation or depression of the metatarsal head. Both the shortening and the position in the transverse plane may be controlled intraoperatively by palpation and by checking under a C-arm (**Fig. 2**). Soft tissue contractures can be relaxed through shortening of the corresponding metatarsal. Sometimes this shortening means that other WOs are needed to balance forefoot propulsive mechanics. In the presence of a second metatarsophalangeal joint (MTPJ) dislocation, surgical shortening of the second metatarsal usually means all lesser metatarsals need shortening WOs, even if they are "healthy" (although nonfunctional) joints (**Fig. 3**). Besides third-rocker metatarsalgia, hammer toe or claw toe, MTPJ dislocation, second-space syndrome, overlapping, and wind-swept toes are also indications for WO. Barouk's

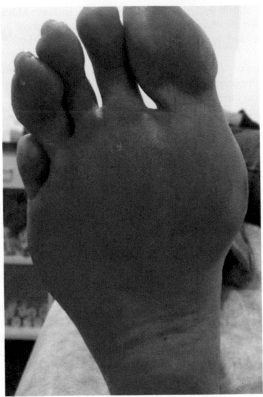

Fig. 1. Third rocker keratoses are plantodistal to the metatarsal heads. Third rocker/propulsive metatarsalgia may benefit from WOs.

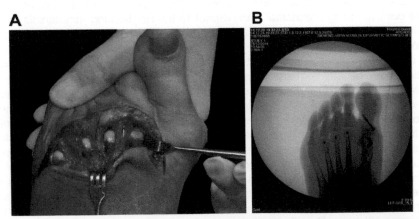

Fig. 2. Dorsal approach for WOs. (*A*) Dorsal Weil exposure allows for visual inspection and palpation of the metatarsal parabola. (*B*) Intraoperative fluoroscopy also allows controlling metatarsal length after WOs.

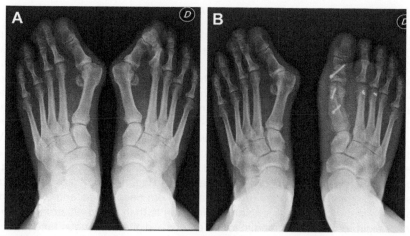

Fig. 3. Restoration of the metatarsal parabola and joint restoration in MTPJ dislocation are indications for WO. (*A*) Preoperative weight-bearing dorsoplantar radiograph showing dislocation of the second MTPJ in the right foot. (*B*) Postoperative radiograph showing restored second MTPJ. WO of the third metatarsal was needed to create a harmonic metatarsal parabola.

concept of "shortening with longitudinal decompression" of the forefoot together with lateral/medial displacement of WO provides soft-tissue relaxation that allows for the correction of the aforementioned deformities.[4,5] Contraindications for WO include second rocker metatarsalgia, osteoporosis, and trophic disturbances.

SURGICAL ANATOMY OF THE LESSER METATARSALS

Metatarsal heads receive blood from epiphyseal, metaphyseal, and diaphyseal vessels.[10,11] In the dorsal aspect of a lesser metatarsal, the *dorsalis pedis* arteries give small metaphyseal capital arteries. In the plantar aspect, the metatarsal is irrigated from a plantar metaphyseal capital artery that arises from the corresponding intermetatarsal artery. WO does not damage this artery and makes necrosis a very unlikely event in this osteotomy.[10,11] As the metaphyseal area is better irrigated, osteotomies should fall within the surgical neck of the metatarsal in order to heal faster. Diaphyseal regions of the bone will take longer healing times and are more prone to nonunion or malunion.

The second metatarsal has only dorsal interosseous muscles and not plantar, which might explain why active plantar flexion is more difficult for the second toe than for the rest of lesser toes.[12] Both the transverse and the sagittal planes have to be taken into account when performing the correct WO. There are variations in both the transverse and the sagittal plane disposition of the metatarsals. In the transverse plane, metatarsal parabola was studied by different investigators.[9,13] The first and second metatarsal should be equal in length, and then decreasing lengths should be 4, 6 and 12 mm from the third to the fifth metatarsals. When a patient presents with this formula (originally or postoperatively) it is very uncommon for them to develop propulsive metatarsalgia. In the sagittal plane, declination with respect to the horizontal plane was found to be around 15° for the second metatarsal, 10° for the third, 8° for the fourth, and 5° for the fifth.[14] So the cuts for WOs should have a progressive dorsoplantar inclination from the second to the fifth metatarsals.

SURGICAL TECHNIQUE WITH TIPS AND PITFALLS

Surgery should be planned in advance by drawing the preoperative template to precisely calculate how many metatarsals should be operated and the amount of shortening needed in each of them.

Popliteal-block anesthesia and a below-the-knee tourniquet are used depending on the surgeon's preference. Surgical approach to the lesser metatarsals may be planned depending on how many osteotomies are needed to achieve the correct metatarsal parabola. Longitudinal incisions over the metatarsals were originally used by Barouk and others.[5] A longitudinal skin incision was used for adjacent metatarsals. Weil used a single curved transverse dorsal incision that offered adequate exposure of lesser MTPJ and was skin-friendly (**Fig. 4**).[15] The incision is deepened through the subcutaneous tissues with special care to avoid damage to the neurovascular structures. Subcutaneous tissues are reflected away from deep fascia and extensor tendons to expose the MTPJ. A longitudinal incision is then made either lateral to the extensor digitorum brevis or medial to the extensor digitorum longus tendon, or between both to expose the capsule. A linear incision will open the capsule and 2 Hohmann retractors help to fully expose the metatarsal head and protect the collateral structures. Excessive stripping of the dorsum of the metatarsal should be avoided. Over time we have become friendlier with the soft tissues around the joint, and less exposure would possibly mean less retraction of dorsal tissues and lower incidence of floating toes. Collateral ligaments should ideally be preserved to maintain lateral and medial stability.

Milimetric corrections in metatarsal osteotomies require appropriate instrumentation. A controlled bone cut to avoid excessive bone resection needs to be performed by using a long thin saw blade (**Fig. 5**). The osteotomy is started 2 mm inferior to the most dorsal aspect of the articular cartilage (intraarticular) and cut orientation should be as much parallel to the ground/weight-bearing plane as possible and at around 25° angle with respect to the shaft of the second metatarsal. The angle of the osteotomy will vary according to the declination angle of the metatarsals, with an increase toward the more lateral rays that are less plantarflexed than the second metatarsal. Orientation also depends on the variations of WO (ie, triple WO). On completion of the osteotomy, the metatarsal head will smoothly shift proximally to a more decompressed position. The "neutral" position of the head will reflect soft tissue relaxation, which

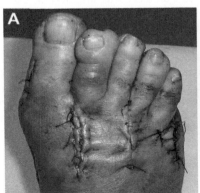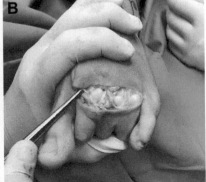

Fig. 4. Surgical approaches for WO may consist of (*A*) longitudinal incisions over the metatarsals or (*B*) a single transverse dorsal incision that allows a more convenient visualization and palpation of the metatarsal heads.

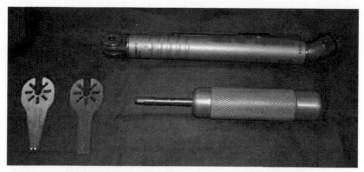

Fig. 5. Small bone power tools and a long thin saw blade are indispensable for WO.

(in most cases) will be coincident with the shortening planned in the preoperative template (unless there is a pathologic contracture of the extensor tendons). A longer metatarsal cut would potentially allow for a "second fixation shot" proximally in case of a pin-screw cut-out through the dorsal aspect of the metatarsal. In a long-cut osteotomy (especially in osteoporotic bone), a Kirschner wire may be inserted proximally to maintain position and the desired shortening before proceeding to fixating the osteotomy distally.

Predrilling of the dorsal cortex of the metatarsal may help in controlling screw or pin insertion and to avoid fracture and cut-out while inserting the implant (Video 1). Plantar pushing of the head dorsally coaptates the fragments. The metatarsal head is held in place with the help of a small curved clamp while introducing the screw or pin with a slow-motion power drill. The most conventional fixation method uses a 2.0 mm twist-off screw driven across the osteotomy plane from dorsal proximal to plantar distal into the plantar condyles of the metatarsal head. Temporary fixation with the use of a small Kirschner wire may be of use to check the desired shortening of the metatarsal under fluoroscopy. As the screw head touches the metatarsal, the thin attachment of the screw to the support will break and fixation may be finished with the screw driver if needed (Video 2). The screw should be placed not too distally so as to prevent contact with the proximal phalanx on maximum dorsiflexion of the toe. The dorsal peak of the osteotomy is smoothed using a small bone rongeur. In most of the adults, a 13 mm twist-off screw will correctly fix the second metatarsal, a 12 mm screw will fix the third, and 11 mm screws will work for the fourth and the fifth metatarsals.

If more than 3 mm of shortening is required, Barouk recommended a "second layer" cut to produce elevation and to compensate for the plantar flexion associated with big displacements of the metatarsal head.[5] Maceira's modification of the WO is an evolution of WO and will be described later.

Several other fixation methods have been proposed for WO.[16] Initially, Weil used the Weil and Schwartz Snap of Compression Pin (S.O.C. Pin) to fix the osteotomy.[5] It provided fragment compression and had a self-rupture at the support of the pin. Kirschner wires, either smooth or threaded, also give adequate stability to an already stable osteotomy.[5] Barouk and the French Pied Innovation Group developed a twist-off screw, a compressive self-tapping and flat-headed device that soon became popular in Europe (**Fig. 6**).[5] Cannulated or solid screws from 1.6 mm to 2.4 mm have also been used to fix WO. No significant differences have been found between lag screw fixation and self-drilling screws.[17] Absorbable pin fixation has also led to good clinical results with a low incidence of complications.[18] A comparative study of WO with and without fixation showed no significant clinical differences.[19]

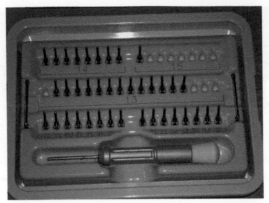

Fig. 6. Twist-off screws for WO as developed by Barouk and the French Pied Innovation Group.

Intraoperative X-ray control is advisable to check metatarsal length/parabola. Tourniquet is released and careful hemostasis is done by coagulation of small vessels before skin closure with absorbable 2-0 suture. Toe/forefoot bandaging is then done with lesser toes in plantar flexion.

POSTOPERATIVE CARE

Primary bone fixation is obtained by implants through the osteotomy plane. Secondary bone fixation is obtained by the correct postoperative toe plantar flexion bandaging. The dressing should control edema and plantarflex the toes and will possibly contribute to the reduction of dorsal soft tissue retraction and floating toes. The authors routinely use postoperative bandaging for 4 weeks postoperatively with changing of bandage weekly. The patient is advised to wear a postoperative shoe and not to "toe-off." Postoperative shoe helps patients to maintain partial weight bearing for the first 4 weeks postoperatively. Immediate weight bearing is allowed as tolerated.

The patients are taught and encouraged to passively plantarflex their toes, leg crossed over knee, in the first 8 weeks postoperatively. The role of passive plantar flexion in floating toes following WO has been studied.[20] Other postoperative regimes include the use of dorsal locking orthosis for the prevention of floating toes after WO with satisfactory results.[21]

EVOLUTION FROM SIMPLE WEIL TO TRIPLE WEIL

In the mid-1990s, Ernesto Maceira (senior author), an orthopedic surgeon based in Madrid (Spain), realized that the modification of the shape of the distal region of a metatarsal after WO might induce changes that contributed to stiffness and floating toes. Maceira developed a modification of the WO, now known as triple (three-step-cut) WO, to try to avoid those complications.[7,8]

This modification sought to recreate a more anatomic metatarsal after the osteotomy, while preserving the relative length and position of the interossei musculature in relation to the center of rotation at the MTPJ. The three-step approach respects the biomechanics of the MTPJs. The shape and integrity of the cartilage of the metatarsal head are not altered with this extraarticular technique. The shortening is done coaxial to the shaft.

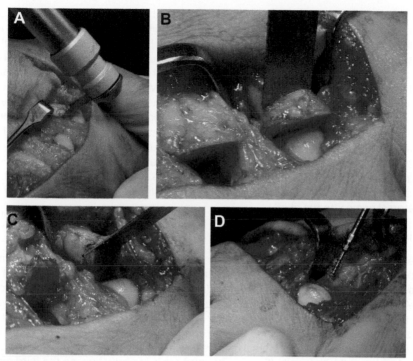

Fig. 7. Triple-cut WO by Maceira. (*A*) First oblique cut (extraarticular). (*B*) Second dorsoplantar cut with the planned amount of shortening in the dorsal aspect of the metatarsal. (*C*) Third cut at the edge created by the second cut is oblique and parallel to the first cut. (*D*) Fixation of the osteotomy with a twist-off screw.

Three cuts are made to shorten (and not simultaneously plantarflex) the metatarsal (**Fig. 7**). The first oblique cut is initiated just at the proximal border of the dorsal metatarsal cartilage extraarticularly. The orientation of the cut is more inclined than the standard WO and plantarly penetrates the distal cortex just proximal to the capsular insertion of the MTPJ. The amount of planned shortening is measured over the distal dorsal aspect of the metatarsal metaphysis and the second cut is performed, from dorsal to plantar, perpendicular to the ground. The second cut creates a new edge at which another oblique cut is made parallel to the first cut. This third cut will produce a bone cylinder of the distal metaphyseal-diaphyseal region of the metatarsal allowing shortening without simultaneous plantar displacement of the head (Video 3). Unlike the conventional WO, the shape of the metatarsal head is anatomically preserved with the triple WO.

In 2001, Trnka and colleagues[22] reported on their in vitro research of WO that it was impossible to complete the osteotomy plantar-proximally with an orientation of the blade less than 25° with respect to the metatarsal diaphysis. The average inclination angle of the second metatarsal is 15°, so the final inclination of the osteotomy should be 10° at minimum and it would be impossible to perform the cut parallel to the ground. This inclination would implicate a plantar flexion effect of the WO. The more shortening needed the more plantar flexion will result from WO. Plantar flexion associated with shortening would be even more notorious in the third, fourth, and fifth metatarsals whose inclination angles are less than 15°. When shortening of the metatarsal is 3 mm or more, there is metatarsal head plantar displacement, which could potentially be clinically relevant by transforming a third rocker metatarsalgia into a second rocker metatarsalgia.[7,8] With contradictory results, the effect of shortening and simultaneous plantar displacement of the metatarsal head has been studied by other investigators in sawbone models and in cadaveric studies with no proven clinical evidence.[23,24] Trnka and colleagues[22] also reported that plantar flexion of the metatarsal head produces a change in the axis of rotation of the MTPJ. In a conventional WO dorsal interosseous muscles would change their function from acting in a position inferior to the axis (plantar flexion of the digit) to a position superior to the axis (dorsiflexion of the digit—floating toe expected). This explanation has been used to explain the high incidence of floating toes after WO.[25] However, the authors believe the causes underneath floating toes after WO may be multifactorial and other factors explained throughout the text would possibly have an influence in this condition. Triple WO addresses potential mechanical drawbacks of conventional WO via shortening of the metatarsal coaxial to the shaft.

VARIATIONS OF WEIL OSTEOTOMY

Several modifications of the WO have been described in the past 15 years, the most important being the triple WO that has been previously presented.[7,8] Other modifications include coronal plane displacement (medial or lateral sliding) to correct crossover/overriding toes.[26,27] Medial or lateral translation of the metatarsal head is indicated for the correction of abduction or adduction deformities of the toes in transverse plane conditions such as the second space syndrome.[1,7,8] The second toe is in adduction so the second metatarsal head is translated medially one-third or half of its width to correct the deformity (Fig. 8). The third toe is in abduction, so the third metatarsal head is translated laterally in the same way.

The "second layer" modification by Barouk included a second cut parallel to the conventional cut in order to compensate for the plantar flexion associated with shortening/decompression larger than 3 mm.[5] This variant of WO may be useful in the management of second rocker metatarsalgia. In a cadaveric study, Grimes and Coughlin used a thick saw blade to offset a portion of the plantar displacement of the head that occurs with WO.[28] They concluded that the use of a 2-mm thick saw blade (vs the conventional 1-mm saw blade) was recommended for shortening of more than 5 mm or with plantar inclination of less than 19°, and a thicker saw blade should be considered for the treatment of second rocker plantar keratosis. The results of this study showed that a 2-mm thick saw blade could resemble the effect of a triple WO and a thicker saw blade that of a "second layer" WO.

The "tilt up" variant of the WO makes a wedge with the apex located distally and the base proximally in a bid to create metatarsal head elevation in cases of second rocker metatarsalgia due to prominent plantar condyles. The "tilt down" variant consists in making the opposite wedge.

The percutaneous distal mini-invasive metatarsal osteotomy (DMMO) is a purely extraarticular technique that resembles WO. A distal dorsal to proximal plantar cut is performed and no fixation is used. Metatarsal length is supposed to be set automatically on weight bearing of the foot in the postoperative period.[29] DMMO may also be considered a variant of WO.

COMPLICATIONS

Complications of conventional WO include floating toes, recurrence, transfer metatarsalgia, delayed union, nonunion, and malunion. In a literature review of 1131 WOs,

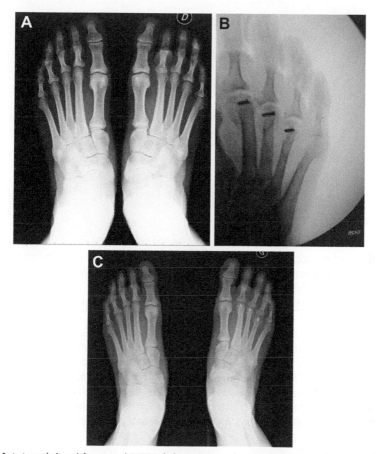

Fig. 8. Metatarsalgia with second MTPJ dislocation and second space syndrome in the right foot. (*A*) Preoperative weight-bearing dorsoplantar radiograph. (*B*) WOs with medial translation of the head of the second metatarsal. (*C*) Postoperative radiograph showing restored second MTPJ, toe deformity, and metatarsal parabola.

Highlander and colleagues[30] found an overall occurrence of floating toes in 36% of cases. Recurrence was reported in 15% of patients and transfer metatarsalgia in 7% of cases. Delayed union, nonunion, and malunion had a collective incidence of 3% of the cases. No differentiation was made between WO and triple WO.

Floating Toes

The most frequent complication of WO is the floating toe, in up to 36% of cases (**Fig. 9**).[30] There is a mechanical explanation for this complication. The reduction of the plantar flexor mechanism tension associated with the retraction of the dorsal structures during the healing process of the surgical procedure may be the cause for this negative evolution. A "floating" toe has inadequate ground contact and sometimes an excess of pressure is developed under the metatarsal head. There is high propensity for the MTPJ to develop hyperextension deformity.[31] Some floating toes are not symptomatic and cause no rubbing with shoewear. But in case of a painful floating toe either because of the contracture of the MTPJ or because of rubbing with shoewear (or both), a full capsular incision and release along with extensor tendon

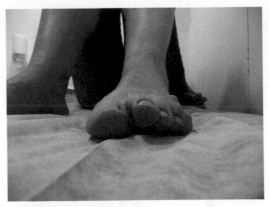

Fig. 9. Floating toes after WOs.

lengthening and postoperative strapping in plantar flexion may restore toe position. A careful surgical technique with minimal soft tissue dissection and triple WO combined with postoperative splintage (plantar flexion bandages) and postoperative plantar flexion stretching exercises minimize the incidence of floating toes after WO.[32,33]

Recurrence

Recurrence of subluxation or dislocation of the MTPJ may be due to undercorrection (not adequate shortening) or scarring of the dorsal soft tissues producing dorsal translation and extension of the joint. Joint stiffness is directly linked to the amount of shortening and may also be due to postoperative fibrosis, biomechanical impairment of the intrinsic muscles, or reaction to implants used for fixation. Management of recurrence usually means a new WO or triple WO aimed to restore joint space.

Transfer Metatarsalgia

Poor technique may result in inadvertent lowering or elevation of the metatarsal heads. In case of abnormal lowering a second-rocker metatarsalgia under the impaired metatarsal may ensue. In case of abnormal elevation of the metatarsal head a second-rocker metatarsalgia may develop under the neighbor lesser metatarsal. Abnormal relative shortening of one metatarsal with respect to the neighboring lesser metatarsal may generate a third rocker/propulsive transfer metatarsalgia. A combination of frontal and sagittal plane malalignment may be present in some patients, so a combination of

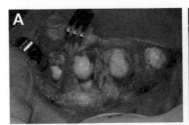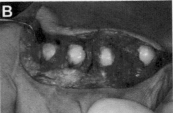

Fig. 10. Combination of frontal and sagittal plane malaligment following metatarsal surgery. (*A*) Second metatarsal is plantarly displaced and longer than the neighboring metatarsals. (*B*) Correction with a triple Weil osteotomy with harmonic frontal and sagittal plane alignment.

triple WOs with tilt-up osteotomies may be needed to restore forefoot alignment and biomechanics (**Fig. 10**).

Delayed Union, Nonunion, Malunion

Poor surgical technique may result in inadvertent lowering or elevation of the metatarsal heads following WO. Cut-out of the fixation screw may also facilitate nonunion of the osteotomy (**Fig. 11**). Malrotation of the metatarsal head is usually the result of an oblique cut in WO and may be managed with a wedged-osteotomy to restore the correct alignment of the metatarsal head.

RESULTS AND OUTCOMES

Most clinical studies have showed good to excellent results after WO. Trnka and colleagues[34] reviewed the correction of subluxed or dislocated MTPJs treated with the Helal osteotomy and WO. After the Helal procedure, only 8/21 joints were reduced, but 21/25 subluxed or dislocated joints were reduced after WO.[34] The same investigator reported excellent results in 21 patients (42 WO) for the treatment of dislocated lesser metatarsal joints.[35]

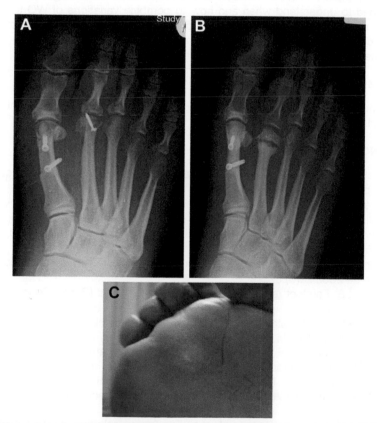

Fig. 11. Nonunion of a WO may lead to transfer metatarsalgia. (*A*) Screw cut-out after WO. (*B*) Screw removal and development on nonunion with shortening and elevation of the metatarsal head. (*C*) Six months postoperatively second rocker keratosis under the third metatarsal and metatarsalgia is congruent with altered forefoot mechanics after failed WO.

Beech and colleagues[36] studied the outcomes of WO in 51 patients (89 procedures) with 80% of patients satisfied. A subgroup of patients who underwent WOs along with a first metatarsal procedure also scored well in terms of function and pain.

WO and triple WO have been reported to be effective procedures in the management of propulsive (third rocker) metatarsalgia.[37,38] Good to excellent long-term results have been reported in 70% to 100% of patients treated with conventional WO.[25,39] Hofstaetter and colleagues[25] showed 88% good results for WO with an 8-year follow-up.

Several papers have compared the outcomes of Weil osteotomies with mini-invasive distal metatarsal metaphyseal osteotomies (DMMO).[40–42] No significant differences were found in terms of range of motion and patient satisfaction. Extraarticular DMMO is supposed to minimize postoperative stiffness.[29] However, a longer period of postoperative edema might be the cause of a longer postoperative recovery after DMMO.[43]

Rheumatoid feet may also benefit from WO as long as there is a correct control of the disease and joints are not severely affected.[44–46]

In view of these results, WO is an effective and safe procedure for the treatment of third rocker/propulsive metatarsalgia. Triple WO may even show better results than those referred to conventional WO, but more studies are needed to fully understand the limits of triple WO in the management of propulsive metatarsalgia. More studies are needed to understand when and how to combine variations of WO to achieve the best mechanical environment for the forefoot with metatarsalgia. Complications may be controlled with a judicious preoperative planning, with a meticulous surgical technique, and with the correct postoperative care.

SUPPLEMENTARY DATA

Supplementary data related to this article can be found online at https://doi.org/10. 1016/j.fcl.2019.08.009.

REFERENCES

1. Pascual-Huerta J, Arcas-Lorente C, García-Carmona FJ. The Weil osteotomy: a comprehensive review. Rev Esp Podol 2017;28(2):e38–51.
2. Maceira E. Aproximación al estudio del paciente con metatarsalgia. Revista Pie Tobillo 2003;17:14–29.
3. Perry J. Gait analysis: normal and pathological function. Thorofare (NJ): Slack; 1992.
4. Espinosa N, Maceira E, Myerson MS. Current concept review: metatarsalgia. Foot Ankle Int 2008;29(8):871–9.
5. Barouk LS. Forefoot reconstruction. 1st edition. France (Paris): Springer-Verlag; 2003.
6. Barouk LS. Weil's metatarsal osteotomy in the treatment of metatarsalgia. Orthopade 1996;25:338–44.
7. Maceira E, Fariñas F, Tena J, et al. Analysis of metatarsophalangeal stiffness following Weil osteotomies [in Spanish]. Rev Med Cir Pie 1998;12:35–40.
8. Espinosa N, Myerson MS, Fernandez de Retana P, et al. A new approach for the treatment of metatarsalgia: the triple Weil osteotomy. Tech Foot Ankle Surg 2009; 6:254–63.
9. Maestro M, Besse JL, Ragusa M, et al. Forefoot morphotype study and planning method forforefoot osteotomy. Foot Ankle Clin N Am 2003;8:695–710.
10. Yamada T, Gloviczki P, Bower TC, et al. Variations of the arterial anatomy of the foot. Am J Surg 1993;166:130–5.

11. Tonogai I, Hayashi F, Tsuruo Y, et al. Distances from the deep plantar arch to the lesser metatarsals at risk during osteotomy: a fresh cadaveric study. J Foot Ankle Res 2018;11:57.
12. Pisani G. Trattato de chirurgia del piede. 1st edition. Torino (Italy): Minerva Médica; 1990.
13. Tanaka Y, Takakura Y, Kumai T, et al. Radiographic analysis of hallux valgus. A two-dimensional coordinate system. J Bone Joint Surg Am 1995;77(2):205–13.
14. Weijers R, Kemerink G, van Mameren H, et al. The intermetatarsal and metatarsal declination angles: geometry as a source of error. Foot Ankle Int 2005;26(5): 387–93.
15. Dalal R, Mahajan RH. Single transverse dorsal incision for lesser metatarsophalangeal exposure. Foot Ankle Int 2009;30:226–8.
16. Jex T, Wan CJ, Rundell S, et al. Analysis of three types of fixation of the Weil osteotomy. J Foot Ankle Surg 2006;45:13–9.
17. Rabenhorst BM, Smith MP, James CR, et al. Biomechanical comparison of lag screw versus self-drilling screw fixation of oblique metatarsal osteotomy. Foot Ankle Int 2011;32(8):811–7.
18. Morandi A, Dupplicato P, Sansone V. Results of distal metatarsal osteotomy using absorbable pin fixation. Foot Ankle Int 2009;30(1):34–8.
19. García-Fernández D, Gil-Garay E, Lora-Pablos D, et al. Comparative study of the Weil osteotomy with and without fixation. Foot Ankle Surg 2011;17:10–7.
20. Perez HR, Reber LK, Christensen JC. The role of passive plantar flexion in floating toes following Weil osteotomy. J Foot Ankle Surg 2008;47(6):520–6.
21. Godoy-Santos AL, Diniz Fernandes T, Luzo C, et al. Effectiveness of the dorsal thermoplastic locking orthosis to prevent floating toes in postoperative follow-up of Weil osteotomies: pilot study. Foot Ankle Spec 2014;7(5):356–62.
22. Trnka HJ, Nyska M, Parks BG, et al. Dorsiflexion contracture after the Weil osteotomy: results of cadaver study and three-dimensional analysis. Foot Ankle Int 2001;22:47–50.
23. Melamed EA, Schon LC, Myerson MS, et al. Two modifications of the Weil osteotomy: analysis on sawbone models. Foot Ankle Int 2002;23(5):400–5.
24. Lau JT, Stamatis ED, Parks BG, et al. Modifications of the Weil osteotomy have no effect on plantar pressure. Clin Orthop Relat Res 2004;421:194–8.
25. Hofstaetter SG, Hofstaetter JG, Petroutsas JA, et al. The Weil osteotomy: a seven year follow-up. J Bone Joint Surg 2005;87:1507–11.
26. Bevernage BD, Deleu PA, Leemrijse T. The translating Weil osteotomy in the treatment of an overriding second toe: a report of 25 cases. Foot Ankle Surg 2010;16: 153–8.
27. Klinge SA, McClure P, Fellars T, et al. Modification of the Weil/Maceira metatarsal osteotomy for coronal plane malalignment during crossover toe correction: case series. Foot Ankle Int 2014;35:584–91.
28. Grimes J, Coughlin M. Geometric analysis of the Weil osteotomy. Foot Ankle Int 2006;27(11):985–92.
29. Redfern D. Treatment of metatarsalgia with distal osteotomies. Foot Ankle Clin N Am 2018;23:21–33.
30. Highlander P, von Herbulis E, Gonzalez A, et al. Complications of the Weil osteotomy. Foot Ankle Spec 2011;4:165–70.
31. Phisitkul P. Managing complications of lesser toe and metatarsophalangeal joint surgery. Foot Ankle Clin N Am 2018;23:145–56.
32. Espinosa N, Brodsky JW, Maceira E. Metatarsalgia. J Am Acad Orthop Surg 2010;18(8):474–85.

33. Migues A, Slullitel G, Bilbao F, et al. Floating-toe deformity as a complication of the Weil osteotomy. Foot Ankle Int 2004;25:609–13.
34. Trnka HJ, Mühlbauer M, Zettl R, et al. Comparison of the results of the Weil and Helal osteotomies for the treatment of metatarsalgia secondary to dislocation of the lesser metatarsophalangeal joints. Foot Ankle Int 1999;20:72–9.
35. Trnka HJ, Gebhard C, Mühlbauer M, et al. The Weil osteotomy for treatment of dislocated lesser metatarsophalangeal joints: good outcome in 21 patients with 42 osteotomies. Acta Orthop Scand 2002;73(2):190–4.
36. Beech I, Rees S, Tagoe M. A retrospective review of the Weil metatarsal osteotomy for lesser metatarsal deformities: an intermediate follow-up analysis. J Foot Ankle Surg 2005;44:358–64.
37. Khurana A, Kamadabande S, James S, et al. Weil osteotomy: assessment of medium term results and predictive factors in recurrent metatarsalgias. Foot Ankle Surg 2011;17:150–7.
38. Perez Muñoz I, Escobar-Antón D, Sanz-Gómez TA. The role of Weil and triple Weil osteotomies in the treatment of propulsive metatarsalgia. Foot Ankle Int 2012;33: 501–6.
39. Vandeputte G, Dereymaeker G, Steenwerckx A, et al. The Weil osteotomy of the lesser metatarsals: a clinical and pedobarographic follow-up study. Foot Ankle Int 2000;21:370–4.
40. Yeo NE, Lob B, Chen JY, et al. Comparison of early outcome of Weil osteotomy and distal metatarsal mini-invasive osteotomy for lesser toe metatarsalgia. J Orthop Surg (Hong Kong) 2016;24:350–3.
41. Johansen JK, Jordan M, Thomas M. Clinical and radiological outcomes after Weil osteotomy compared to distal metatarsal metaphyseal osteotomy in the treatment of metatarsalgia-a prospective study. Foot Ankle Surg 2019;25(4):488–94.
42. Rivero-Santana A, Perestelo-Pérez L, Garcés G, et al. Clinical effectiveness and safety of Weil's osteotomy and distal metatarsal mini-invasive osteotomy (DMMO) in the treatment of metatarsalgia: A systematic review. Foot Ankle Surg 2018. https://doi.org/10.1016/j.fas.2018.06.004.
43. Henry J, Besse JL, Fessy MH. Distal osteotomy of the lateral metatarsals: a series of 72 cases comparing the Weil osteotomy and the DMMO percutaneous osteotomy. Orthop Traumatol Surg Res 2011;97(Suppl):S57–65.
44. Barouk LS, Barouk P. Joint-preserving surgery in rheumatoid forefoot preliminary study with more-than-two-year follow-up. Foot Ankle Clin 2007;12:435–54.
45. Krause FG, Fehlbaum O, Huebschle LM, et al. Preservation of lesser metatarsophalangeal joints in rheumatoid forefoot reconstruction. Foot Ankle Int 2011;32: 131–40.
46. Trieb K, Hofstaetter SG, Panotopoulos J, et al. The Weil osteotomy for correction of the severe rheumatoid forefoot. Int Orthop 2013;37(9):1795–8.

Distal Minimally Invasive Metatarsal Osteotomy ("DMMO" Procedure)

Olivier Laffenêtre, MD[a,b], Anthony Perera, MBChB, FRCS(Orth)[c,*]

KEYWORDS

- Keyhole foot surgery • Minimally invasive • Metatarsalgia • Metatarsal osteotomy

KEY POINTS

- Lesser metatarsal osteotomy is a useful technique for the management of failed conservative treatment of metatarsalgia.
- The ideal procedure enables a 3-dimensional correction that is stable and respects the metatarsal cascade.
- The percutaneous approach enables this procedure to be performed in a minimally invasive manner.

INTRODUCTION

Lesser ray osteotomies are one of the best treatments for metatarsalgia after failure of nonoperative treatment. They allow for potential displacement of the distal capital fragment in 3 dimensions, thus modifying the weight bearing on the metatarsal head, in order to alter the functional impact across all the metatarsal heads.

Lateral metatarsal osteotomies have 2 potential difficulties; first is to respect the anterior arch of the metatarsal heads in the coronal and sagittal plane and secondly to obtain a sufficient stability in order to maintain the desired correction.

In general, the more proximal a procedure is the less stable it is. In addition, osteotomies oriented from dorsal-distal to plantar-proximal are more stable than those that are vertical or perpendicular to the metatarsal axis or those oriented from plantar-proximal to dorsal-distal.

The recent arrival of percutaneous surgery as a surgical tool is still a problem, as there is a paradox between a very large use on lesser rays, with very good or excellent clinical results regularly reported, and the lack of literature on the subject.

Disclosure Statement: Both are members of GRECMIP.
[a] Foot & Ankle Institut, 136 bis rue Blomet, Paris 75015, France; [b] University Medico-Surgical Foot Center, Pellegrin University Hospital, Place Amélie Raba-Léon, Bordeaux 33076, France; [c] Spire Cardiff Hospital, Croescadarn Road, Cardiff, Wales CF 23 8XL, UK
* Corresponding author.
E-mail address: anthony@footandankleuk.com

THE PERCUTANEOUS TOOL

It seems relevant to introduce the percutaneous tool, which is not so different today from the arthroscopy of the 80s as a target of much criticism. The use of this tool first appeared in the United States under the influence of the "father of the minimally invasive incision in foot surgery" Morton M Polokoff (1908–2001) about 60 years ago, and its use has been developed by North American podiatrists. The level of technical development and the quality of the publications was insufficient for this to make significant impact until, thanks to S Isham MD, DPM, in the 1980s when this surgery was rigorously taught and began to be credible.[1]

It was subsequently introduced into Europe by De Prado in Spain in 1994. He established along with Golanó the surgical and anatomic bases essential for a safe and reproducible practice.[2] It was then further developed in France from 2002, under the aegis of the Research Group and Study in Minimally Invasive Surgery of the Foot (GRECMIP).[3]

The incision is created with a mini-blade ("beaver blade") for the soft tissues and a power rotatory burr for the bony procedures. This technique is performed through a working incision, as small as 1 to 3 mm long and thus without direct visualization of the underlying target structures. Instead it is guided by intraoperative fluoroscopy (**Figs. 1** and **2**).

There is a false assumption that it is difficult to perform minimally invasive surgery, as some procedures sometimes are very different from those performed in a conventional open approach and that this is further compounded by the absence of visual control (other than fluoroscopy). In this respect percutaneous surgery is quite close to arthroscopic surgery.

Concerning lesser ray osteotomies, the main challenge remains the ability to balance sufficiently correction of the plantar hyperpressure while at the same time preserving a harmonious metatarsal arch in the anteroposterior and frontal planes, by avoiding a transfer metatarsalgia.[4]

The absence of osteosynthesis far from being a disadvantage of this approach is in fact the main asset of this procedure, providing the ability to allow "self-adjustment" of the metatarsal heads according to the distribution of the ground reaction forces. However, this does require some control in order to prevent excessive movement and the osteotomies are initially controlled by a dressing, which is removed generally after 2 weeks, and replaced by cohesive strips (**Fig. 3**) for a few more weeks. During this time walking and thus loading of the metatarsal heads is encouraged, as this facilitates normalization of the pressure under the metatarsal heads.

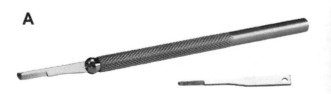
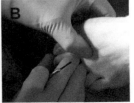

Fig. 1. (*A*) Beaver holder and its two 1- and 3-mm blades. (*B*) The use of a 3-mm blade to perform DMMOs.

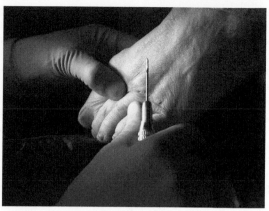

Fig. 2. A power rotatory burr is required to perform DMMOs.

TECHNIQUE
Surgical Procedure (Described for Distal Metatarsal Minimal Invasive Osteotomy Surgery on the Left Foot by a Right-Handed Surgeon)

De Prado{DePrado:2003vn}{DePrado:2016jx} then GRECMIP is a research organisation and described this independently of De Prado.[5,6]

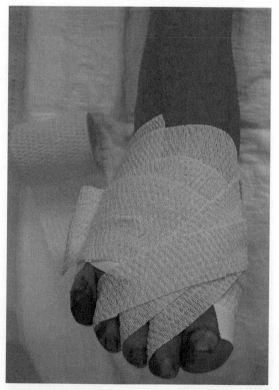

Fig. 3. After the first dressing at 2 weeks, cohesive elastic strips can be used to maintain the direction of the operated toes.

This is an extraarticular osteotomy where the correction occurs slightly more proximally than the Weil osteotomy and begins 2 to 3 mm from the articular surface in the neck area, in an extraarticular location (**Fig. 4**). A 2 × 12 mm Shannon burr is required for the osteotomy.

For surgery on a left foot by a right-handed operator, the top of the metatarsal head must first be palpated with the left thumb. Then at this level in the interspace on the right side of the head (ie, lateral side for the left foot) the operator performs a 2-mm incision, preparing a path for the burr by using a periosteal elevator and positioning obliquely the burr at a 45° angle to the metatarsal axis, against the neck. This can be done by feel, using the instrument to move along the flare on the proximal part of the head onto the neck.

This area of bone must be firmly rasped (excursion of no more than 1 cm) to peel off the soft tissues, thus preserving them. It allows a precise location of the distal point on the neck corresponding to the beginning of the head. Once the surgeon reaches it, he/she leans the burr by 45° to the metatarsal axis.

Before cutting, the head is clamped between the left thumb and the forefinger.

The correct positioning of the burr may be checked with a C-arm at the beginning, but with experience, this will not be necessary. Identification of the transition from the flare of the head to the narrower neck is reliable achieved by feel alone.

The osteotomy with the motorized burr begins with the section of the lateral cortex, moving plantar and medial, and ends with the section of the dorsal cortex. This is done by pivoting in a rotational movement from the point of skin entry. This involves a supination of the wrist through 90°. The burr thus comes to almost lie flat on the foot at 90° to the metatarsal axis in the anteroposterior plane (**Fig. 5**).

To avoid a lateral translation, it is necessary, depending on the side, right or left of the foot, to finish the cut with an angle of 135° or 45°, respectively with respect to the metatarsal axis, again for a right-handed operator (**Fig. 6**). By producing a somewhat oblique cut in the dorsoplantar projection, the lateral cortex is slightly longer than the medial cortex, thus producing a buttress to lateral displacement, as this is the natural direction for drift.

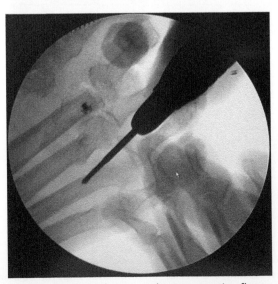

Fig. 4. Location of the burr in the neck area under peroperative fluoroscopic control.

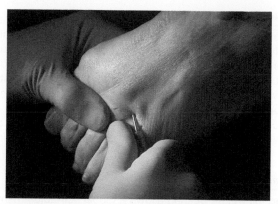

Fig. 5. Position of the burr at a 90° angle from the metatarsal axis at the end of the cut.

It is very important to mobilize the toe in the metatarsal axis to make sure that the metatarsal heads can move together with full weight bearing by mobilizing periosteal adhesions that could prevent the shortening and elevation of the distal fragment. This is performed using the straight elevator through the incision to release the soft tissues.

Planning for DMMO does not require the same considerations as for open surgery, and therefore, it is generally necessary to perform osteotomy on the second, third, and fourth, even if the fourth metatarsal is less overloaded and thus usually asymptomatic. The addition of the fourth metatarsal does seem to permit a more harmonious alignment of the metatarsal heads in relation to one another. A nonpropulsive or static metatarsalgia, which appears during the second rocker when the entire foot contacts the ground under the gastrocnemius eccentric contraction control (in case of a correct lenght of this muscle), is probably the best indication for 2/3/4 DMMOs.

Furthermore, another excellent indication is a propulsive metatarsalgia that appears during the third rocker when only the forefoot contacts the ground and is more in relation with an excess of metatarsal lengths.

The main rule is never to perform an isolated DMMO and to be very careful by performing only 2.

This is why different evolutions of DMMOs were designed and particularly in such a case, the distal intracapsular minimally invasive osteotomy (DICMO).

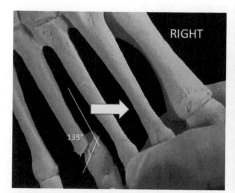
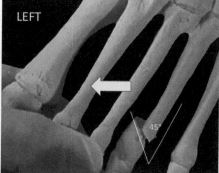

Fig. 6. Direction of the final cut by 135° (*right* foot) and 45° (*left* foot) to avoid a lateral displacement.

Postoperative Dressings

DMMOs are not often done in isolation and are often associated with a hallux valgus deformity and lesser toe deformity, which is also usually into valgus. Postoperative dressings therefore must help to control this drift into valgus but can also help to control the metatarsal heads that may drift into valgus if multiple DMMOs have been performed. It can be difficult when the second to fourth or fifth are done together. The natural drift is lateral and therefore dressings such as gauze and crepe are used to hold the toe in a straight alignment while permitting natural motion of metatarsophalangeal (MTP) and proximal interphalangeal joints.

Postoperative Management

An immediate and full weight bearing allows a global self-adjustment, the metatarsal heads aligning with one another and the ground reaction force. It is preferable for this to be done in a more physiologic postoperative flat shoe. The patient needs to be aware that the foot will be more swollen and sore; this can be much more so than if a percutaneous hallux valgus is done in isolation.

The shoe needs to be worn for 3 until the swelling reduces sufficiently for normal but comfortable footwear. However, range of motion of the MTP joints is encouraged from immediately after surgery.

EVOLUTIONS
Distal Intracapsular Minimally Invasive Osteotomy

DMMO has the potential for a significant displacement by the self-adjustment. Furthermore, this technique can be associated with more pain and edema, which disappears only when the bone healing is obtained.[7–9]

Therefore, in some cases an intraarticular osteotomy called a DICMO that is closer to a Weil can be proposed instead of a DMMO. Unlike DMMO, it can be performed in isolation, especially in case of a painful instability of the second or third metatarsal.

The cut is more stable, allowing a simple elevation of the width of the 2-mm burr with a millimeter of shortening or none. After a medial approach with a beaver blade respecting the extensor system laterally and then penetrating the capsule, the 2 × 12 mm Shannon burr approaches the top of the articular surface. Following a 45° angle it will cross the plantar cortex behind the joint. A scan of the burr then makes it possible to cut the bone while remaining within the capsular limits, which will avoid any major displacement, particularly lateral or medial (**Fig. 7**).

Distal Oblique Metatarsal Minimal Invasive Osteotomy

The DMMO allows a maximum shortening of only 5 mm, therefore a new osteotomy has been developed that allows more significant shortenings: the distal oblique metatarsal minimal invasive osteotomy (DOMMO).

The direction of the burr may be convergent toward the first ray (**Fig. 8**) or on the contrary, divergent. This allows the surgeon to guide the displacement and may exceed 1 cm. The bone approach, medial or lateral, depending on the desired effect, is metaphyseal from dorsal-distal to plantar-proximal. No osteosynthesis is required and the longer the cut is the higher the expected shortening is.

This osteotomy can be mixed with a Weil, which will be used for a dislocated ray (ie, when major shortening is needed). This is the principle of such a hybrid surgery that avoids an extensive Weil procedure to the other lesser rays, leading to much better functional results (**Fig. 9**).

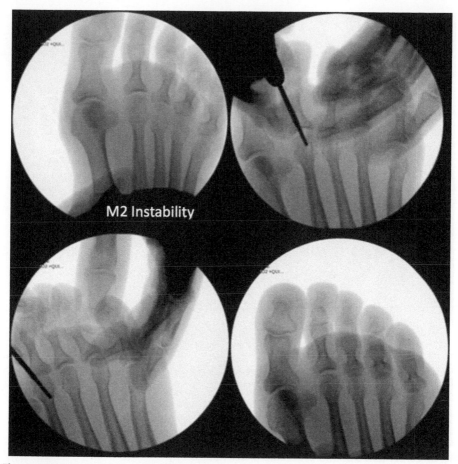

Fig. 7. DICMO procedure under fluoroscopy.

KNOW THE RESULTS AND BENEFITS: STATE OF THE ART

Many osteotomies have been advocated for the treatment of metatarsalgia; however, for some time now the Weil osteotomy{Barouk:1996ud} has been established as the procedure of choice around the world.

The ability to correct the parabola to accepted norms{Maestro:2003ua} and further-more the ability to control this correction with fixation was seen as key to the success of this operation. Moreover, the fixation permitted earlier mobilization. Studies comparing the Weil with the earlier Helal osteotomy{Helal:1975vj}, an unfixed distal metatarsal osteotomy, strongly supported these arguments{Trnka:1999 hg}.

These experiences have therefore drawn unfavorable comparisons of the DMMO with the Helal osteotomy. However, the DMMO is a very different philosophy. Firstly, the Helal osteotomy was angled in the opposite direction and thus uncontrolled eleva-tion was a major problem resulting in a high risk of transfer metatarsalgia. Secondly, the fact that it was an open operation further destabilized head and also created more scar tissue.

Because experience with the Weil has increased, there has been a growing aware-ness of its failings. It is good at shortening the metatarsal but not as good at elevating

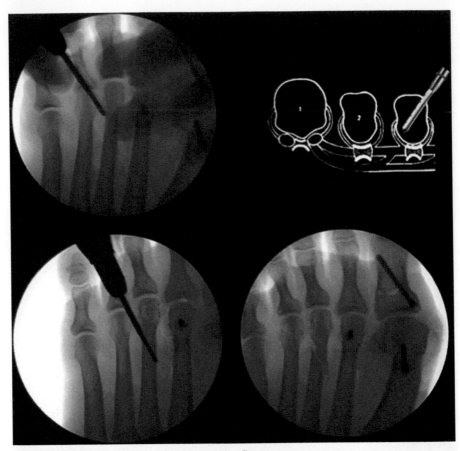

Fig. 8. Convergent DOMMO procedure under fluoroscopy.

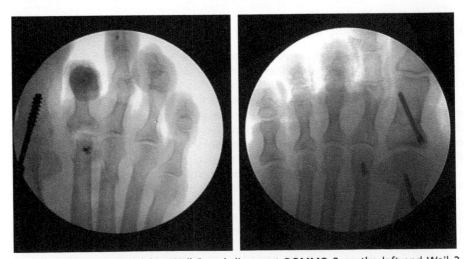

Fig. 9. Hybrid surgeries mixing Weil 2 and divergent DOMMO 3 on the left and Weil 2, convergent DOMMO 3 and DMMO 4 on the right.

the head. Studies have shown that in fact there is a risk of plantarising the head instead and that this may be implicated in the floating toe deformity{Trnka:2001fr}. Other complications include stiffness and arthrofibrosis{Reddy:2018el}, and these risks are likely to be influenced by the fact that there is a significant soft tissue approach and that the osteotomy is intraarticular.

Interest has therefore grown in alternatives to this such as the unfixed Weil osteotomy{GarciaFernandez:2011kf}. However, the DMMO is an extraarticular osteotomy done in a percutaneous manner with minimal soft tissue dissection that permits elevation as well as shortening. The concern has been that it seems to be a step back to the Helal osteotomy, but the direction of the osteotomy and the soft tissue preservation means that it is better at controlling excessive dorsiflexion.

The lack of fixation is key to the mode of action of a DMMO, but there has been concern that this may result in uncontrolled displacement. However, a comparative study{Henry:2011gk} of 39 patients treated with DMMO and 33 patients treated with Weil with the head placed at a predetermined position showed that the postoperative correction was similar. In this study, the overall outcomes as scored by the American Orthopedic Foot and Ankle Society score were similar and the incidence of recurrent metatarsalgia was similar. The key difference was that the risk of stiffness was less for DMMO (normal movement or slight stiffness was 62% vs 43%). The price for this was that at 3 months there was more swelling in DMMO patients. All the DMMOs went on to unite, but delayed union was an issue compared with the fixed Weil.

Similar results have been shown in other papers with comparison to Weils {Yeo:2016gn}{Thomas:2017fq} and case series{Wong:2013fd}. In Magnan's series {Magnan:2017ex}, 88% of patients had excellent outcomes. However, they were also able to demonstrate excellent range of motion and also a low rate of complications. However, there is a learning curve and it is important that the burr is handled with care, as nonunion and necrosis can occur{Krenn:2018eh}.

In one British study{Haque:2016es} of 30 patients assessed by Manchester–Oxford Foot Questionnaire, Visual Analogue Scale, and radiological measures excellent results were shown. They also demonstrated that there was a low risk of infection. However, there was 1 nonunion and 1 patient who had a second and third DMMO who went on to develop transfer metatarsalgia to the fourth metatarsal and which then required correction. However, there is little other support for prophylactic osteotomy of the fourth metatarsal in these circumstances.

Despite the lack of fixation, malunion is very unusual. The commonest cause for this is that the osteotomy has been made too proximally and has been performed through the shaft rather than the metaphysis. Usually in these circumstances the metatarsal becomes shorter and/or more dorsal than desired. Orthotics are certainly worth trying, as the malunion is generally not significant if it occurs; however, if it is then revision surgery may be required. The easiest technique is to revise the other metatarsals that will then reset to the level of the malunited one. This is however not always possible, in which case one must decide whether an open revision is required.

In an exceptional case of nonunion, 2 options are possible:

- First, considering that a lack of immobilization is the main cause of it, the nonunion must be stabilized on either side, by wirering the metatarsals to its neighbors for 6 weeks; weight bearing is allowed thanks to a flat shoe that needs to be worn for this time. This procedure was described by Diebold[10] before the arrival of percutaneous surgery (Diebold-91) and has always led a complete healing in our hands (**Fig. 10**).

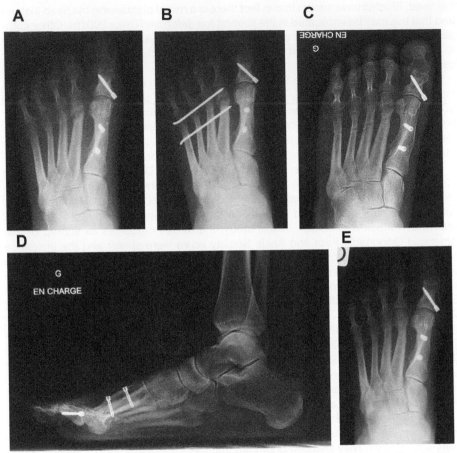

Fig. 10. Nonunion of the DMMO 2 after a 2-year follow-up (*A*) treated according the Diebold's method (*B*). Aspect 10 weeks after the removal of both wires (*C*, *D*) and 2 years after the revision (*E*).

- Secondly, considering that nonunion is the consequence of a lack of pressure under one or more metatarsal heads, due to a plantar situation and precocious bone healing of one metatarsal, de Prado suggests performing new DMMOs around the nonunion. Postoperative care is the same as in the first surgery.

SUMMARY

The knowledge of different types of metatarsal osteotomies allows to determine the ideal indication to each clinical situation, in order to obtain the most reliable result. Regarding the treatment of metatarsalgia, percutaneous distal metatarsal osteotomies provide results comparable to those obtained by Weil osteotomy at the cost of fewer complications and much less technical difficulties. Its use to treat metatarsal pathologies has become essential. The percutaneous tool is an alternative that offers for lesser rays a different concept based on self-adjustment. Its interest will have to be evaluated in retrospect.

However, the use of such an osteotomy does not allow to treat all cases, so in GRECMIP we have imagined some evolutions of it, which can enlarge the indications of the percutaneous technique to treat metatarsalgia.

REFERENCES

1. Ischam S. The Reverdin-Isham procedure for the correction of hallux valgus – a distal metatarsal osteotomy procedure. Clin Podiatr Med Surg 1991;8:81–94.
2. De Prado M, Ripoll PL, Golanó P. In Cirugia percutanea del pie. Tecnicas quirurgicas, indicaciones, bases anatomicas. Barcelona (Spain): Masson; 2003.
3. Laffenêtre O, Golanó P, GRECMIP. Introduction à la chirurgie mini-invasive du pied et de la cheville : pourquoi, quand, comment ? Académie Chir, e-mémoire 2010;9(1):52–60.
4. Feibel JB, Tisdel CL, Donley BD. Lesser metatarsal osteotomies. A biomechanichal approach to metatarsalgia. Foot Ankle Clin 2001;6:473–89.
5. De Prado M, Ripoll PL, Golanó P, et al. Cirurgia percutanea del pie. Barcelona (Spain): Masson SA; 2003. p. 167–82.
6. Coillard JY, Laffenêtre O, Cermolacce C, et al. Traitement chirurgical des métatarsalgies statiques par technique percutanée. In: Masson, editor. Chirurgie de l'avant-pied 2ème édition, Cahiers d'enseignement de la SOFCOT. Amsterdam: Elsevier; 2005. p. 153–7.
7. Salinas Gilabert JE, Lajara Marco F, Ruiz Herrera M. Distal percutaneous osteotomy in the treatment of lesser ray metatarsalgia. Rev Esp Cic Ortop Traumatol 2009;53(3):192–7.
8. Darcel V, Villet L, Chauveaux D, et al. Prise en charge de métatarsalgies statiques par ostéotomies distales percutanées : suivi prospectif de 222 pieds. In: Monographie AFCP, vol. 5. Montpellier (France): Sauramps; 2009. p. 229–42.
9. Henry J, Besse JL, Fessy M-H, AFCP. Distal osteotomy of the lateral metatarsals : a series of 72 cases comparing the Weil osteotomy and the DMMO percutaneous osteotomy. Orthop Traumatol Surg Res 2011;97(6 Suppl):S57–65.
10. Diebold P-F, Daum B. le pied post traumatique. In: Hérisson C, Claustre J, et al, editors. Simon. Paris: Masson; 1991. p. 8–15.

State of the Art in Lesser Metatarsophalangeal Instability

Sudheer C. Reddy, MD

KEYWORDS

- Metatarsophalangeal joint instability • Plantar plate tear • Lesser toe tendon transfer
- Lesser toe arthroscopy • Metatarsal osteotomy

KEY POINTS

- Clinical evaluation remains the best method for diagnosis of MTP instability
- Recent trends have demonstrated a shift in surgical treatment toward anatomic repair of deficient structures
- Adjunctive techniques such as arthroscopy and minimally invasive surgery have also been increasingly used to address instability
- Use of synthetics has also gained in popularity to augment anatomic repair

INTRODUCTION

Lesser metatarsophalangeal (MTP) instability remains a clinically challenging condition for both the clinician and patient. Perhaps in no other condition are the results as visible and apparent as with lesser toe surgery. The clinician must take into the account not only coronal and sagittal plane and even rotational deformities of the lesser toes, but also consider more global conditions that could affect stability such as metatarsus adductus. Specific imaging modalities tailored to imaging of the lesser toes have also been used to aid the clinician in diagnosis. Advancements in tendon transfers, osteotomies, and repair of native supporting structures have all been made in recent years.[1] Deciding which procedures to use, and when, can be a complex task. Much of the recent attention and advancements have been made in addressing plantar plate disorder given its role in MTP instability. Additional methods of tendon transfers and osteotomies, both new and modifications of existing ones, have also been used. Each treatment plan, however, should be individualized to the patient, and proper preoperative evaluation is essential. Managing patient expectations is paramount because complications such as digital stiffness, persistent swelling, and pain can remain even in a well-aligned toe.

Department of Orthopaedic Surgery, Shady Grove Orthopaedics, Adventist Health Care, George Washington School of Medicine, 9601 Blackwell Road, Rockville, MD 20850, USA
E-mail address: sreddy8759@yahoo.com

Foot Ankle Clin N Am 24 (2019) 627–640
https://doi.org/10.1016/j.fcl.2019.08.007
1083-7515/19/© 2019 Elsevier Inc. All rights reserved.

foot.theclinics.com

CLINICAL EXAMINATION

A thorough history should be taken when assessing for lesser MTP instability, with care taken to assess for the duration and location of pain, inciting and alleviating factors, and treatment methods used. Pain is typically the predominant complaint of early MTP instability without loss of dorsal or collateral restraint, which will be localized to the MTP joint and often during the third rocker phase of gait.[2] The pain is often gradual in onset.[2,3] Less commonly, a traumatic event can initiate instability.[4] A history of injections is important, given the adverse effect of multiple cortisone injections on stability (**Fig. 1**). Patients may also note the onset of malalignment of the toes, difficulty with shoewear, or swelling. Additional pertinent historical information includes the presence of autoimmune arthropathies, peripheral vascular disease, and neurologic or congenital conditions that could influence treatment plans.

Examination of a patient with MTP instability should begin with a weight-bearing assessment of alignment. Hindfoot alignment is important to note as well as that of the midfoot, because more proximal malalignment can affect overall stability of the MTP joints. Hallux valgus or varus can further influence MTP stability and affect treatment (**Fig. 2**). Further assessment should evaluate for tenderness along the MTP joint or plantar plate, presence of any callosities, and loss of alignment of the toes. Callosities can be present along the metatarsal head, proximal or distal interphalangeal (IP) joint, or along the terminal aspect of the toe. Patients may note impingement or drifting of the involved toes. The reducibility of the lesser toe deformity is also important to assess because this can dictate treatment. In a prospective evaluation, Nery and colleagues[4] noted that the second MTP joint is most frequently affected (64% of the time), with the third and fourth less commonly affected (32% and 4%, respectively). The location of pain is also critical to note because conditions of instability tend to be localized to the joint itself, typically in the base of the proximal phalanx, but can be difficult to distinguish from signs of an interdigital neuroma such as interdigital pain. In approximately 20% of cases, an interdigital neuroma and MTP instability can coexist.[5] Diagnostic lidocaine injections can assist in diagnosis.

Thompson and Hamilton[6] originally described the use of the MTP drawer test to assess for stability, whereby both the metatarsal head and respective proximal phalanx are independently stabilized and a vertically directed force is applied to the base of the proximal phalanx. The degree of laxity and pain elicited when performing this maneuver often indicate the integrity of the plantar plate and can alert the examiner to the extent of instability.[4,7,8] Klein and colleagues,[3] in a study of 90 patients,

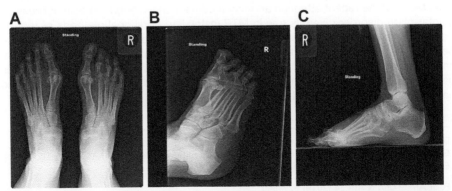

Fig. 1. Preoperative anteroposterior (AP) (*A*), oblique (*B*), and lateral (*C*) images demonstrating right second MTP dorsal dislocation following multiple cortisone injections.

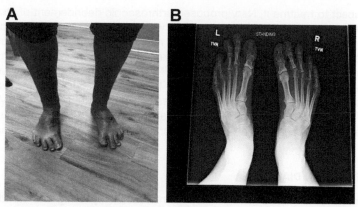

Fig. 2. (*A*) Clinical image of a patient with right hallux varus, varus instability of MTP 2, 3 in setting of metatarsus adductus. (*B*) AP view of foot.

noted that a positive drawer sign coupled with a gradual onset of pain and pain localized to the metatarsal head was present in 95% of patients with a plantar plate tear. The paper pull-out test, whereby a piece of paper is placed under the involved toe, is an additional examination that can alert the clinical to subtle instability. An ability to grasp the paper with the affected toe indicates intact digital purchase. Inability to do so can indicate the loss of intrinsic stability and function.[9,10]

CLASSIFICATION

Much attention has been devoted recently to the evaluation and classification of MTP instability to help guide treatment. Nery and colleagues[4] and Coughlin's group[11] proposed clinical and anatomic grading schemes. Anatomic grading schemes have focused on the morphology of the plantar plate.

Clinical staging of lesser MTP instability[4]

Grade	Alignment
0	Prodromal phase, no instability
1	Mild deformity, web-space deviation
2	Moderate deformity with toe elevation and medial/lateral deviation
3	Severe deformity with toe elevation, overlap, flexible hammertoe deformity
4	Dislocation of toe, crossover toe, fixed hammertoe deformity

Anatomic staging of plantar plate tears (anatomic grading system)[4,12]

Grade	Description
0	Plantar plate/capsular attenuation
1	Transverse distal tear <50% of width Midsubstance tear <50%
2	Transverse distal tear >50% Midsubstance tear >50%
3	Transverse/longitudinal extensive tear ± involvement of collateral ligaments; T tear/V tear
4	Cruciform-type tear with buttonhole of metatarsal head (MTP dislocation)

With respect to treatment, Nery proposed arthroscopic debridement of stage-0 lesions, distal metatarsal shortening osteotomy with plantar plate repair, and collateral ligament reefing for stages 1 to 3, and distal metatarsal shortening osteotomy with flexor-to-extensor transfer for stage-4 disorder. In their series of 22 patients, Nery and colleagues[4] noted that the second MTP joint was most commonly affected, with grade-3 tears most frequently observed. Lateral deviation of the toe was infrequently noted. Of note, 30% of patients had residual hyperextension at the MTP joint with 63% being able to achieve plantigrade alignment and ground purchase. They noted that stage-3 and stage-4 lesions were less likely to achieve plantigrade alignment.

ADVANCEMENTS IN DIAGNOSIS

Advancements in diagnosis have primarily centered on improving and standardizing imaging modalities to aid in visualization of the plantar plate, collaterals, and surrounding structures. With respect to MRI, a common protocol used in imaging the forefoot includes a dedicated extremity coil with the following sequences: (1) coronal short-axis T1-weighted spin-echo images; (2) fat-suppressed T2-weighted images in the coronal short-axis, sagittal, and axial long-axis planes[13] (**Fig. 3**) Contrast enhancement with gadolinium can further aid in diagnosis.[14] Fluid interposition is considered to pathognomonic of a plantar plate tear, but is not always present.[13,15,16] Use of the anatomic grading system has been shown to improve the diagnostic accuracy of MRI. In a series of 35 patients for whom MRI findings were correlated to direct arthroscopic visualization, the anatomic grading system was found to improve the sensitivity and overall accuracy of both experienced and novice radiologists in evaluating plantar plate tears.[12] Yamada and colleagues[13] concluded that routine use of 1.5-T MRI is useful and sufficient when performed in patients with clinical suspicion of MTP instability. Using the aforementioned protocol and when considering any change in the morphology of the plantar plate, MRI was found to have a sensitivity of 97% and specificity of 100% in diagnosing tears. Furthermore, the presence of pericapsular fibrosis around the base of the proximal phalanx extending into the intermetatarsal space (pseudoneuroma sign) and the plantar plate-proximal phalanx distance were independent predictors of plantar plate tears. With respect to distance from the plantar plate to proximal phalanx, a cutoff value of 0.275 cm was found to have a sensitivity of 65% and specificity of 90% in diagnosing tears.[13]

Though not a first-line modality in the evaluation of lesser MTP instability, the use of weight-bearing computed tomography (CT) imaging can be helpful in assessing the metatarsal cascade and osseous morphology. Coronal images can be viewed to

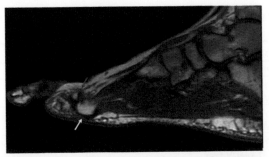

Fig. 3. Sagittal coronal proton density–weighted image demonstrating a dorsal third MTP dislocation (*red arrow*) with retraction of the plantar plate (*yellow arrow*).

analyze the relative orientation of the metatarsal heads for possible elevation or declination. Instances of osteotomy malunion, osteonecrosis, and osteoarthritis can be discerned and aid the clinician, particularly in instances of failed surgery when the diagnostic accuracy of MRI can be hindered by metal artifacts (**Fig. 4**).

SURGICAL TREATMENT
Role of Arthroscopy

Arthroscopy has started to emerge as a method for diagnosing and treating early stages of MTP instability. Advantages include smaller incisions with less morbidity relative to more traditional open approaches and potentially a faster recovery. Indications for arthroscopy include its use as a diagnostic tool, synovectomy, evaluating and treating MTP instability, addressing chondral lesions, and loose body removal.[17–19]

Setup for Lesser Metatarsophalangeal Arthroscopy

- Patient is placed supine on the operating room (OR) table with the foot at the end of the bed. An ankle or calf tourniquet may be used for hemostasis[17–19]
- A toe strap attached to a distractor can aid in visualization
- A standard 1.9- or 2.7-mm 30° arthroscope is sufficient for examination along with small joint probes, curettes, awls, and 2.0-mm shaver. Small radiofrequency ablators can also be used to address plantar plate disorder (stage-0 lesions).
- Standard dorsomedial and dorsolateral portals are marked equidistant from the extensor digitorum longus (EDL) tendon (approximately 4–5 mm) along the plane of the MTP joint or slightly distal (**Fig. 5**). The joint is insufflated with 2 mL of saline.
- A no. 11 blade is used to incise the skin with a blunt hemostat used to dissect down and perforate through the capsule via a nick-and-spread technique. One must be careful along the medial aspect of the second MTP joint when making the dorsomedial portal because of the proximity of the dorsal digital branch of the deep peroneal nerve.[17]
- The arthroscope is inserted with 100% continuous flow and 30 mm Hg of fluid pressure. Manual or mechanical distraction can be used, but one must be careful of excess distraction caused by neuropraxia.
- Standard examination involves the sequential evaluation of the 3 sections of the MTP joint:[17,20]
  - *Medial gutter*: medial proper and accessory collateral ligaments, Medial bundle of plantar plate

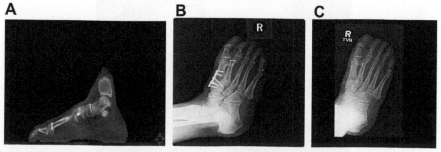

Fig. 4. (*A*) Sagittal weight-bearing CT image of a Weil distal metatarsal osteotomy malunion s/p prior plantar plate repair. The patient was unable to extend her second toe postoperatively. (*B*) Oblique weight-bearing image. (*C*) The patient underwent a dorsal closing-wedge corrective osteotomy to restore alignment and active extension of the toe.

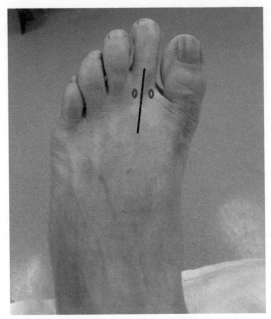

Fig. 5. Clinical image demonstrating standard dorsomedial and dorsolateral portals for lesser MTP arthroscopy.

- ○ *Lateral gutter*: lateral proper and accessory collateral ligaments, Lateral bundle of plantar plate
- ○ *Central joint*: medial and lateral bundles of plantar plate; synovial recess
- Diagnostic arthroscopy is performed in similar fashion to the hallux MTP joint or other small joint arthroscopy using a combination of probes, shavers, and biters (**Fig. 6**). Radiofrequency ablators can be used in grade-0 lesions but should be done so sparingly because of the increased risk of thermal necrosis and potential chondrolysis given the small volume of the joint.[21] Nery and colleagues,[17] in a cadaveric study, demonstrated that standard MTP arthroscopy was more than

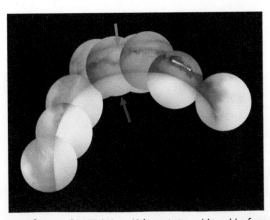

Fig. 6. Panoramic view of second MTP joint with metatarsal head in foreground (*red arrow*) and base of proximal phalanx at top of picture (*green arrow*). Probe is inserted through dorsolateral portal with a lateral transverse plantar plate tear. (*Courtesy of* Caio Nery, MD.)

90% accurate in visualizing and identifying the corresponding structures in each compartment Radiofrequency ablation has been demonstrated to restore subtle instability in grade-0 and grade-1 lesions in combination with a distal metatarsal osteotomy.[22]

Applications of Arthroscopy in Lesser Metatarsophalangeal Instability

Arthroscopic-assisted double plantar plate tenodesis

In addressing plantar plate disorder, arthroscopy has been used to aid in suture passage through the plantar plate. Lui and LiYeung[19] used an arthroscopically assisted modified double plantar plate tenodesis to correct 7 clawtoe and 3 crossover-toe deformities with no evidence of recurrence at final follow-up. An initial arthroscopic release of the joint is performed using a small periosteal elevator or biter. In this technique, for a varus crossover toe deformity, a #1 PDS suture is passed through the medial and lateral aspects of the plantar plate using a straight needle under arthroscopic guidance. A proximal incision is made along the dorsum of the diaphysis of the metatarsal. The sutures are then brought proximally via a hemostat deep to the flexor tendon sheath and tenodesed to the extensor digitorum brevis (EDB). Correction of the deformity can be achieved by variable tensioning of the sutures. In the case of a clawtoe deformity, the suture limbs are brought along the medial and lateral aspect of the metatarsal shaft and sutured to the EDL.[19] Patients were kept non–weight bearing for 2 weeks in a bulky Jones dressing, followed by weight-bearing walking in a wooden sandal for 4 weeks with free mobilization of the toe before resuming regular shoewear.

Arthroscopic direct plantar plate repair

A direct plantar plate repair can also be performed arthroscopically, as described by Nery. Initial debridement and detachment of the plantar plate can be performed with use of a shaver and a Beaver blade with care taken to avoid injury to the underlying flexor tendons. Suture passage can then be facilitated via the Arthrex Viper (Arthrex, Naples, FL), which can simultaneously pass and retrieve sutures through the plantar plate. The viewing portal can then be switched and the remaining limb can be passed through the opposite part of the plantar plate, such that a horizontal-type mattress suture can be placed. Alternatively, the passing suture can be looped on itself to create a luggage-tag type configuration. Percutaneous drill holes are then created within the base of the proximal phalanx, with a suture passer used to pass the sutures to the dorsum of the phalanx, similarly to the open approach. A mosquito is then used to retrieve the sutures and tie them on the dorsum of the phalanx, with care taken not to entrap the EDL.[23] This approach is currently in its infancy and, although outcome data are unavailable, it seems to be a viable treatment option in early-stage disorder **(Fig. 7)**.

Role of Soft-Tissue Procedures

Plantar plate repair

Both dorsal and plantar approaches have been advocated for repairing the plantar plate.[2,10] Advantages of the dorsal approach include the ability to visualize intraarticular disorder, address concomitant disorder (hammertoe deformity, collateral instability), or perform a metatarsal osteotomy as needed. Disadvantages include the limited visualization of the plantar plate, and dorsal contracture with possible floating toe deformity. Sufficient exposure of the plantar plate can be achieved through a sequential release of the collateral ligaments and the plantar plate without the absolute need for an osteotomy.[20] A plantar approach permits easier visualization of the

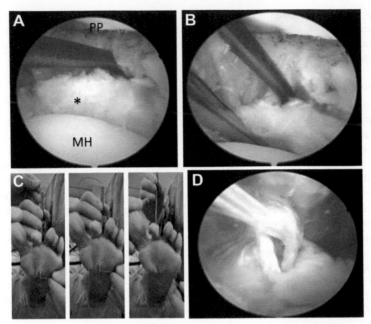

Fig. 7. Steps in arthroscopic plantar plate repair. (*A*) Takedown and mobilization of plantar plate (*asterisk*). (*B*) Suture passer passed through plantar plate. (*C*) External view of suture passage. (*D*) Completed suture passage through plantar plate (luggage-tag configuration). MH, metatarsal head; PP, plantar plate. (*Courtesy of* Caio Nery, MD.)

abnormality without the need to perform an osteotomy but with the potential for injury to the neurovascular bundles and the presence of a plantar scar.[2]

- Dorsal approach (preferred approach) (**Fig. 8**)
  - The patient is placed supine at the end of the OR table with use of an ankle or calf tourniquet for hemostasis.
  - The author prefers a web-space incision to avoid the possibility of a dorsal contracture, although a dorsal or crossover incision can also be used. The interval between the EDL and EDB is developed, exposing the metatarsal head.
  - The decision to perform a distal metatarsal osteotomy is made, depending on the metatarsal cascade.[24,25] A pin-pin distractor (Hintermann) is placed using Kirschner wires in the base of the proximal phalanx and metatarsal head.
  - The plantar plate is then inspected with partial transverse tears completed. Sutures are then passed medially and laterally through the plate with a double-row horizontal mattress configuration preferred by the author.
  - The pin-pin distractor is then removed, and the sutures are passed through the base of the proximal phalanx in a diagonal fashion and secured on the dorsum of the phalanx with the MTP joint in 20° of plantarflexion.
- Plantar approach
  - A web-space incision is typically used with care taken to avoid injury to the digital neurovascular bundle. Exposure of the plantar plate is accomplished by retraction of the flexor tendons.
  - Direct repair can then be performed via suture anchor or bone tunnel fixation.

In their prospective series of 22 patients (40 MTP joints) treated through a combination of a dorsal plantar plate repair with distal metatarsal osteotomy, Nery

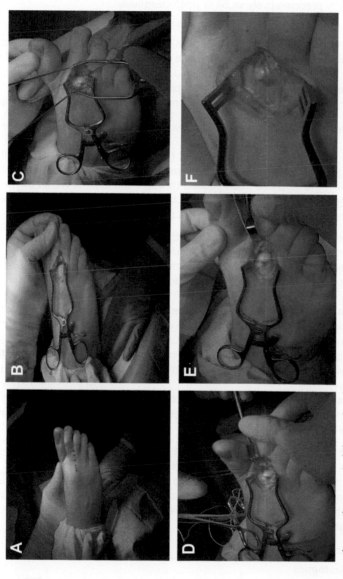

Fig. 8. Steps in open plantar plate repair. (*A*) Initial web-space incision. (*B*) Exposure of the plantar plate. (*C*) Suture passer passed through plantar plate. (*D*) Suture passage through plantar plate. (*E*) Suture passage through proximal phalanx. (*F*) Completed repair. A distal metatarsal osteotomy was not performed.

and colleagues[4] noted an improvement in American Orthopedic Foot and Ankle scores (AOFAS), with grade-1 and grade-2 lesions performing the best overall. Residual hyperextension of the toe was most likely in grade-3 and grade-4 lesions. Flint and colleagues[10] evaluated a larger prospective series of 97 patients (138 plantar plate tears) and noted an overall improvement in pain and AOFAS at 12 months postoperatively. There was a marginal improvement in patients being able to pass the paper pull-out test (42% preoperatively vs 54% postoperatively).

Collateral ligament repair

The role of isolated collateral ligament repair is limited in the overall algorithm of MTP instability. The fan-shaped accessory collateral ligament confers greater dorsal stability in relation to the proper collateral, given its direct attachment to the plantar plate.[26] It should primarily be used as an adjunctive procedure when a plantar plate repair, tendon transfer, or osteotomy is performed, primarily in grade-1 or grade-2 tears.

Tendon transfer (extensor digitorum brevis, extensor digitorum longus, flexor tendon)

Advancements with respect to tendon transfer have primarily revolved around the use of synthetic augmentation of existing procedures. In a variation of the EDB transfer for coronal instability, the EDB has been passed through drill tunnels within the proximal phalanx and metatarsal neck to recreate the lateral collateral ligament and secured with interference screws (Arthrex, Naples, FL) (**Fig. 9**).[27,28]

Steps in internal brace augmentation of EDB transfer
- A dorsal or web-space–based incision can be used
- The interval between the EDB and EDL is dissected and a capsular release is performed. Collateral ligament and partial plantar plate release can be performed as necessary.[27]
- The EDB should be harvested at the level of the musculotendinous junction to provide enough length for the repair. A Z-lengthening of the EDL is performed.
- For a lateral collateral ligament reconstruction, the EDB is passed from distal-medial to proximal lateral within the proximal phalanx and plantar-lateral to dorsomedial within the metatarsal neck. Fixation is secured with 3 × 8-mm interference screws.
- Similarly, a medial collateral ligament reconstruction can be performed with the passage of the EDB in the opposite direction through the proximal phalanx and metatarsal neck.

With respect to plantar plate insufficiency, flexor tendon transfer remains perhaps the best option for addressing grade-4 lesions (**Fig. 10**). In a recent cadaveric study, flexor digitorum longus tenodesis to the base of the proximal phalanx was demonstrated to restore approximately 50% of the stability to dorsal translation relative to the intact plantar plate, and can be considered an alternative to flexor-to-extensor transfer in stage-4 tears.[29]

Role of Osseous Procedures

Metatarsal osteotomies

Metatarsal osteotomies continue to play a role in addressing lesser MTP instability. Magnan and colleagues[30] reported on the use of the percutaneous distal metatarsal metaphyseal osteotomy to treat stage-1 and stage-2 instability in a series of 57 patients (70 feet). There was noted to be an improvement in the subjective symptoms of pain along the metatarsal heads themselves, and overall satisfaction rate of 90% at a mean follow-up of 45 months. Union rate was noted to be approximately 97%

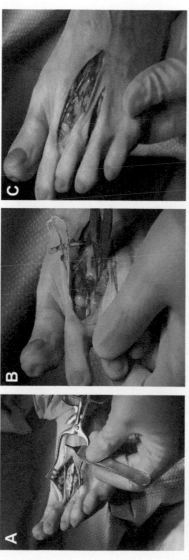

Fig. 9. Steps in EDB transfer for lateral collateral ligament reconstruction: (A) Harvest of EDB. (B) Passage of EDB through drill tunnel in proximal phalanx and through metatarsal neck augmented with FiberTape suture. (C) Completed repair.

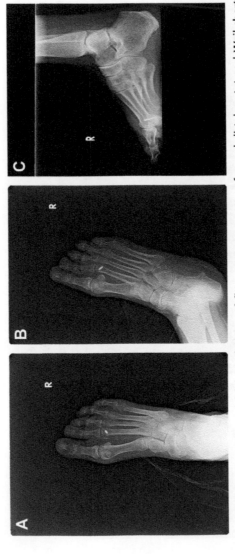

Fig. 10. Postoperative AP (A), oblique (B), and (C) lateral views of flexor-to-extensor transfer and distal metatarsal Weil shortening osteotomy for chronic dorsal second MTP dislocation. **Fig. 1** shows the preoperative images.

at 3 months. The osteotomy was performed using a 2.3-mm Shannon-type burr, starting along the lateral aspect of the metatarsal neck in a dorsal-distal to plantar-proximal direction at a 45° angle to the shaft. Subjects were allowed immediate weight bearing and placed in a toe spica dressing, changed weekly for 6 weeks, to maintain MTP alignment.[30]

SUMMARY

Advancements in treatment of lesser MTP instability have involved the use of arthroscopy, minimally invasive surgery techniques, and synthetic augmentation of existing procedures, with the primary aim of reducing morbidity and facilitating recovery in comparison with traditional approaches. Applicability to specific indications continues to be defined and must be tailored to the specific needs of the patient, with the overall goal of achieving a stable, well-aligned, functional, and painless toe. Although robust clinical data are lacking with respect to the techniques, they are viable options in the appropriate setting.

REFERENCES

1. Nery C, Baumfeld D. Lesser metatarsophalangeal joint instability: treatment with tendon transfers. Foot Ankle Clin N Am 2018;23:103–26.
2. Hsu RY, Barg A, Nickisch F. Lesser metatarsophalangeal joint instability: advancements in plantar plate reconstruction. Foot Ankle Clin N Am 2018;23(1):127–43.
3. Klein EE, Weil L, Weil LS, et al. Clinical examination of plantar plate abnormality: a diagnostic perspective. Foot Ankle Int 2013;34(6):800–4.
4. Nery C, Coughlin MJ, Bamfeld D, et al. Lesser metatarsophalangeal joint instability: prospective evaluation and repair of plantar plate and capsular insufficiency. Foot Ankle Int 2012;33(4):301–11.
5. Coughlin MJ, Schenck RC, Shurnas PS, et al. Concurrent interdigital neuroma and MTP joint instability: long-term results of treatment. Foot Ankle Int 2002;23(11):1018–25.
6. Thompson FM, Hamilton WG. Problems of the second metatarsophalangeal joint. Orthopaedics 1987;10(1):83–9.
7. Kaz AJ, Coughlin MJ. Crossover second toe: demographics, etiology and radiographic assessment. Foot Ankle Int 2007;28:1223–37.
8. Bouche RT, Heit EJ. Combined plantar plate and hammertoe repair with flexor digitorum longus tendon transfer for chronic, severe sagittal plane instability of the lesser metatarsophalangeal joints: preliminary observations. J Foot Ankle Surg 2008;47:125–37.
9. Doty JF, Coughlin MJ. Metatarsophalangeal joint instability of the lesser toes and plantar plate deficiency. J Am Acad Orthop Surg 2014;22(4):235–45.
10. Flint WW, Macias DM, Jastifer JR, et al. Plantar plate repair for lesser metatarsophalangeal joint instability. Foot Ankle Int 2017;38(3):234–42.
11. Coughlin MJ, Schutt SA, Hirose CB, et al. Metatarsophalangeal joint pathology in crossover second toe deformity: a cadaveric study. Foot Ankle Int 2012;33(2):133–40.
12. Nery C, Coughlin MJ, Baumfeld D, et al. MRI evaluation of the MTP plantar plates compared with arthroscopic findings: a prospective study. Foot Ankle Int 2013;34:315–22.
13. Yamada AF, Crema MD, Nery C, et al. Second and third metatarsophalangeal plantar plate tears: diagnostic performance of direct and indirect MRI features

using surgical findings as the reference standard. AJR Am J Roentgenol 2017; 209(2):W100–8.

14. Dinoa V, von Ranke F, Costa F, et al. Evaluation of lesser metatarsophalangeal joint plantar plate tears with contrast-enhanced and fat-suppressed MRI. Skeletal Radiol 2016;45:635–44.

15. Yao L, Cracchiolo A, Farahani, et al. Magnetic resonance imaging of plantar plate rupture. Foot Ankle Int 1996;17:33–6.

16. Yao L, Do HM, Cracchiolo A, et al. Plantar plate of the foot: findings on conventional arthrograpy and MR imaging. AJR Am J Roentgenol 1994;163:641–4.

17. Nery C, Coughlin MJ, Baumfeld D, et al. Lesser metatarsal phalangeal joint arthroscopy: anatomic description and comparative dissection. Arthroscopy 2014;30(8):971–9.

18. Lui TH. Arthroscopy and endoscopy of the foot and ankle: indications for new techniques. Arthroscopy 2007;23:899–902.

19. Lui TH, LiYeung LL. Modified double plantar plate tenodesis. Foot Ankle Surg 2017;23:62–7.

20. Jastifer J, Coughlin M. Exposure via sequential release of the metatarsophalangeal joint for plantar plate repair through a dorsal approach without an intraarticular osteotomy. Foot Ankle Int 2015;36:335–8.

21. Good CR, Shindle MK, Griffith MH, et al. Effect of radiofrequency energy on glenohumeral fluid temperature during shoulder arthroscopy. J Bone Joint Surg Am 2009;91:429–34.

22. Nery C, Raduan FC, Catena F, et al. Plantar plate radiofrequency and Weil osteotomy for subtle metatarsophalangeal joint instability. J Ortho Surg Res 2015; 10:180.

23. Nery C, Baumfeld D, Chan WC, et al. Metatarsophalangeal arthroscopy of the lesser toes. In: Lui TH, editor. Arthroscopy and endoscopy of the foot and ankle. Singapore: Springer Nature Singapore Pte Ltd; 2018. p. 359–94.

24. Maestro M, Besse JL, Ragusa, et al. Forefoot morphology study and planning method for forefoot osteotomy. Foot Ankle Clin 2003;8:695–710.

25. Klinge SA, McClure P, Fellars T, et al. Modification of the Weil/Maceira metatarsal osteotomy for coronal plane malalignment during crossover toe correction: case series. Foot Ankle Int 2014;34:584–91.

26. Barg A, Courville XF, Nickisch F, et al. Role of collateral ligaments in metatarsophalangeal stability: a cadaver study. Foot Ankle Int 2012;33(10):877–82.

27. Ellis SJ, Young E, Endo Y, et al. Correction of multiplanar deformity of the second toe with metatarsophalangeal release and extensor brevis reconstruction. Foot Ankle Int 2013;34:792–9.

28. Haddad SL, Sabbagh RC, Resch S, et al. Results of flexor-to-extensor and extensor brevis tendon transfer for correction of the crossover second toe deformity. Foot Ankle Int 1999;20:781–8.

29. Reilly M, Darvish K, Assari S, et al. Plantar plate reconstruction for stage IV plantar plate tear using flexor tendon tenodesis. Poster Abstract, American Orthopaedic Foot and Ankle Society Annual Meeting. Boston, July 11-14, 2018.

30. Magnan B, Bonetti I, Negri S, et al. Percutaneous distal osteotomy of lesser metatarsals (DMMO) for treatment of metatarsalgia with metatarsophalangeal instability. Foot Ankle Surg 2018;24(5):400–5.

The Role of First Ray Insufficiency in the Development of Metatarsalgia

Angela K. Walker, DO[a],*, Thomas G. Harris, MD[b,c]

KEYWORDS

- Metatarsalgia • First ray insufficiency • Hallux valgus • Metatarsal index

KEY POINTS

- Two theories exist in the development of central or transfer metatarsalgia.
- First, as the severity of hallux valgus increases, there is mechanical overload of the second metatarsal.
- Second, increased relative lesser metatarsal length is thought to contribute to metatarsalgia.
- It is imperative, in the treatment of first ray disorders (hallux valgus or hallux rigidus), to not overshorten the first ray when addressing the first ray pathologic condition.
- Treatment of metatarsalgia in the setting of failed hallux valgus correction can be treated with both conservative and surgical options.

INTRODUCTION

Metatarsalgia generally refers to pain localized to the forefoot. The term transfer metatarsalgia refers to the onset of pain at a different ray than that which is mechanically impaired.[1] There are 3 types of metatarsalgia as described by Espinosa and colleagues.[2] These metatarsalgia include primary, secondary, and iatrogenic. There are 2 different theories that exist in the development of primary metatarsalgia owing to first ray insufficiency. First, in patients with hallux valgus, as the magnitude of the hallux valgus angle (HVA) increases, there is a mechanical overload of the lesser metatarsals. Second, it is thought that increased relative lesser metatarsal length is a factor in the development of metatarsalgia. Iatrogenic causes of first ray insufficiency can also lead to metatarsalgia. Shortening or elevating the first ray during hallux valgus correction can lead to metatarsalgia, as can failing to shorten the second metatarsal during

Disclosures: None.
[a] Orthopedic Surgeons, Inc, 2790 Clay Edwards Drive, Suite 650, Kansas City, MO 64116, USA;
[b] Congress Orthopedic Associates, 800 South Raymond, 2nd Floor, Pasadena, CA 91105, USA;
[c] Foot and Ankle Surgery, UCLA Harbor Medical Center, 1000 W Carson Street, Torrance, CA 90502, USA
* Corresponding author.
E-mail address: drheinen34@gmail.com

Foot Ankle Clin N Am 24 (2019) 641–648
https://doi.org/10.1016/j.fcl.2019.07.001
1083-7515/19/© 2019 Elsevier Inc. All rights reserved.

foot.theclinics.com

surgical correction. In the following, the authors explore the causes of metatarsalgia, specifically related to first ray insufficiency, as well as the various treatment options.

FIRST THEORY: HALLUX VALGUS AND METATARSALGIA

In a "normal" foot, the angle between the first metatarsal and first proximal phalanx (or the HVA) should be less than 20°.[3] When this angle becomes more than 20°, the patient is said to have hallux valgus.[4] According to Coughlin and Jones,[5] hallux valgus can be classified as mild, moderate, or severe, with normal being 15° or less, mild being less than 20°, moderate being between 20 and 40°, and severe being 40° or more. The 1 to 2 intermetatarsal angle (IMA) normally is 9° or less. As the magnitude of hallux valgus increases, this causes a physiologic shortening or insufficiency of the first ray, leading to a mechanical overload of the lesser metatarsals.[6] Foot mechanics are altered in patients with hallux valgus deformity. Deschamps and colleagues[6] found an increased dorsiflexion motion at the hallux during terminal stance. There is a dorsiflexion/adduction moment at the first tarsometatarsal (TMT) joint, which results in a metatarsal head to be more cranially located compared with the other metatarsal head, and a first metatarsal joint to be closer to its neutral position instead of being relatively dorsiflexed. This increased dorsiflexion motion, caused by an earlier onset of the dorsiflexion movement, would therefore be a consequence of the first ray malalignment. They also showed that patients with hallux valgus have a different intersegmental range of motion in the affected foot during barefoot walking when compared with asymptomatic subjects. First TMT instability has also been implicated as a cause of hallux valgus. Dietze and colleagues[7] performed a pedobarographic study on 8 patients that dynamically evaluated the amount of first TMT instability and its relation to hallux valgus and plantar forefoot pressures. Their results showed that increased first TMT joint mobility resulted in a positive significant correlation with maximum force under the second metatarsal, the third metatarsal, and the fourth metatarsal.

SECOND THEORY: METATARSAL LENGTH THEORY

According to Maestro and colleagues,[8] the most common cause of metatarsalgia is a long second metatarsal. Slullitel and colleagues performed a cross-sectional study of 121 consecutive adult patients with non-arthritic hallux valgus and found metatarsalgia present in almost half of the hallux valgus patients. Their findings showed metatarsalgia to have a multifactorial etiology, associated with Achilles shortening, excessive weight, and associated lesser toe deformity. It was not simply related to longer metatarsal length or an increased metatarsal index.[9] A study performed by Kaipel and colleagues[10] theorized that metatarsal length corresponded with plantar-loading parameters under the corresponding metatarsal heads. Their results were somewhat controversial to this theory of the cause of metatarsalgia. They showed that the relative length of the first and third metatarsals did not correlate with the maximal peak pressure or maximal force under the corresponding metatarsal heads.

IATROGENIC CAUSES OF FIRST RAY INSUFFICIENCY AND METATARSALGIA

Iatrogenic metatarsalgia may result from a reconstructive procedure on the foot to address lesser toe abnormality from hallux valgus surgery that has created a shift in plantar pressures to the forefoot.[11] Toth and colleagues[12] followed a series of patients who underwent shortening osteotomy of the first ray for treatment of hallux valgus. The average shortening of the first metatarsal was 3.8 ± 1.8 mm. Positive correlations were found between metatarsalgia of the second through fourth rays and first ray shortening. There was no correlation between fifth ray metatarsalgia and first ray shortening. They concluded that excessive shortening of the first metatarsal should be avoided to decrease the occurrence of postoperative transfer metatarsalgia.

DIAGNOSIS OF METATARSALGIA OWING TO FIRST RAY INSUFFICIENCY

The diagnosis of any condition of the foot starts with a thorough history and physical examination. Important parts to note are any history of trauma, prior surgeries, history of diabetes, or neuropathy. Specifically, in patients with metatarsalgia owing to first ray insufficiency, one must be aware of the following potential findings. Physical examination findings may include plantar keratoses centered under the lesser metatarsal heads, tenderness at the respective metatarsophalangeal (MTP) joint, tenderness or pain with range of motion of the lesser MTP joints, hallux rigidus, hallux valgus, and first TMT instability. A full neurovascular examination, including motor strength testing, sensation to light touch, vibratory sensation, and an evaluation of the dorsalis pedis and tibialis posterior pulses should always be performed. A Silverskiold test should always be performed, because a contracted gastrocnemius complex has been shown to be associated with metatarsalgia. Slullitel and colleagues[9] showed an association between metatarsalgia and the following factors: Achilles shortening, increased body mass index, and lesser toe deformities.

RADIOGRAPHIC FINDINGS

Pertinent radiographic findings to document are metatarsal length and inclinations; also any relative shortening of the first metatarsal should be noted. The severity (if present) of the hallux valgus and IMAs should be measured. The presence of hallux rigidus or arthritic change of the lesser MTP joints should be noted. First TMT instability can be assessed on the lateral radiograph by the presence of plantar gapping, or on the anteroposterior (AP) radiograph by the presence of joint incongruity. Evidence of previous surgeries should be assessed, especially if there has been any shortening of the first ray.

TREATMENT OF METATARSALGIA OWING TO FIRST RAY INSUFFICIENCY
Nonoperative

Management of metatarsalgia is guided toward the cause. "Symptomatic relief can be achieved with physical therapy, shoe modifications, debridement of calluses, and judicious use of corticosteroid injections. When gastrocnemius tightness contributes to metatarsalgia, a stretching program to lengthen the muscles can be instituted."[13] Shoewear modifications can consist of shoes with a wide toe box. Semicustom or custom orthotics can be used, adding metatarsal pads or metatarsal recesses to accommodate areas of pressure on the plantar aspects of the feet.

Operative

Operative management of metatarsalgia owing to first ray insufficiency is tailored to the cause of metatarsalgia. If treatment of hallux valgus is warranted, the appropriate treatment of hallux valgus correction should be undertaken at the surgeon's discretion. The author's preferred treatment of hallux valgus varies depending on the degree of HVA and 1 to 2 IMAs. The treatment algorithm for hallux valgus correction is displayed in **Table 1**.

The differences in plantar pressures after hallux valgus corrective surgery have been studied at length by several different investigators. King and colleagues[14] examined

Table 1 Treatment algorithm for hallux valgus correction			
Hallux Valgus Classification	HVA	IMA	Technique
Mild	25–40	9–13	Distal chevron osteotomy
Moderate	40–50	13–16	Proximal osteotomy ± Akin osteotomy
Severe	40–50	16–20	Proximal or lapidus ± distal osteotomy (consider rotational osteotomy)
First TMT instability	>50	>20	Lapidus procedure or MTP arthrodesis

the differences in plantar forefoot pressures after both distal chevron osteotomy and Lapidus procedures for correction of hallux valgus. Both procedures decreased the pressure under the second metatarsal, but the difference was not significant. The hallux pressure decreased significantly in both procedures. Their Lapidus group showed an overall decrease in the pressure under the second metatarsal head as a percentage of the total forefoot pressure. Cancilleri and colleagues[15] compared distal chevron and triplanar Boc bunionectomy at 24 months. They found that both procedures reduced the hallux and first metatarsal head plantar pressure. The Boc procedure was able to decrease the plantar pressure under the second metatarsal head, but the chevron procedure actually increased the plantar pressure under the second metatarsal head.

In the setting of a relatively long lesser metatarsal, shortening of the metatarsal via several different distal osteotomies can be achieved. Plantar pressures after Weil forefoot osteotomy have been examined in a study by Vandeputte and colleagues.[16] They included 59 metatarsals with pedobarographic evidence of localized increased pressures under the affected metatarsal heads preoperatively. Postoperatively, pressure relief was noted in 48 cases as determined by Harris imprint evaluation. Forty-four of the 59 metatarsals revealed complete resolution of the preoperative plantar callus, indicating plantar pressure relief of the affected metatarsal. In a robotic cadaveric evaluation by Trask and colleagues,[17] a traditional Weil osteotomy performed in the distal to proximal fashion resulted in shortening of the second metatarsal, which thereby decreased the plantar peak pressure and pressure time interval.

In the case of iatrogenic transfer metatarsalgia, there may be shortening of the first ray from a previous procedure, such as hallux valgus correction or from previous first MTP arthrodesis. Lengthening of the first ray may be needed to fully resolve the resultant transfer metatarsalgia. In a series of 6 patients with failed hallux valgus surgery, who had shortening of the first metatarsal and degenerative changes in the first MTP joint, Chowdhary and colleagues[18] describe a technique in which they used a scarf osteotomy with concomitant first MTP joint arthrodesis to allow for lengthening through the first metatarsal. All 6 patients had successful union, returned to full activity, and were completely satisfied with the procedure.

If there is evidence of gastrocnemius contracture and the patient has failed a conservative stretching protocol, consider gastrocnemius recession along with the index procedure as well. Gastrocnemius recession has been indicated in the treatment of secondary metatarsalgia. In multiple studies, surgical gastrocnemius lengthening resulted in increased passive ankle dorsiflexion range of motion (average 14° to 18°), improved function with daily activities, and maintained plantar flexion strength.[19–22]

CASE PRESENTATION

The contributing authors present a case of a 60-year-old woman who initially presented with moderate hallux valgus and plantar pain under the second and third metatarsal heads. Preoperative radiographs show moderate hallux valgus with a 1 to 2 IMA of approximately 13, and an HVA of approximately 32 (**Fig. 1**). The patient is a high-demand, very active patient and opted to not have the second and third preexisting metatarsalgia addressed along with the hallux valgus correction. The patient initially underwent left distal chevron osteotomy, Akin osteotomy, and modified McBride procedure (**Fig. 2**). Approximately 9 months after the index procedure, the patient complained of worsening pain under the second and third metatarsal heads. It was at this point that the patient opted to have second and third Weil osteotomies performed.

DISCUSSION

In the management of metatarsalgia owing to first ray insufficiency, 2 main theories exist. First, in patients with hallux valgus, as the magnitude of hallux valgus increases, there becomes an overload on the lesser metatarsals leading to metatarsalgia. Second, an overall increased relative length of the second metatarsal leads to metatarsalgia. Both of these theories have been tested in the literature.

Slullitel and colleagues[9] examined the relative length of the first and second metatarsals. They defined the feet as minus, equal, and plus. The minus feet had a short first metatarsal compared with the second metatarsal. Equal feet had similar length, and the plus feet had a long first metatarsal. They actually found an inverse relationship in the case of the metatarsal index. They found no significant correlation between metatarsalgia and HVA, 1 to 2 IMA, foot arch type, and metatarsus adductus. Dreeben and colleagues[23] tested the plantar loading parameters of patients treated by dorsal wedge osteotomy compared with those of asymptomatic feet. The patients with metatarsalgia had increased maximal peak pressure and increased plantar flexion of the metatarsal heads of the symptomatic rays. The dorsiflexion osteotomy led to a substantial decrease of maximal peak pressure and an improvement in symptoms in the metatarsalgia group. However, they found no correlation between the length of the metatarsals and plantar loading parameters or symptoms.

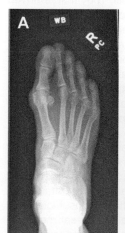
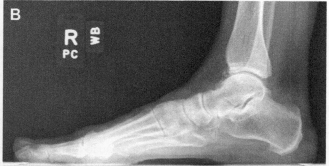

Fig. 1. (A, B) Preoperative standing AP and lateral radiographs show moderate hallux valgus with relatively long second and third metatarsals.

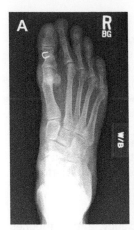
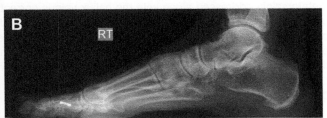

Fig. 2. (*A, B*) Postoperative standing AP and lateral radiographs show correction of hallux valgus with persistent, relatively long second and third metatarsals.

Another study performed by Kaipel and colleagues[10] also examined the relative length of metatarsal compared with the maximal peak pressure and maximal force on the plantar aspect of the foot. They found that relative length of the first and third metatarsals (compared with the second metatarsal) did not correlate with maximal peak pressure and maximal force. Maximal force under the first metatarsal head was decreased in the metatarsalgia group. There was no difference in the maximal peak pressure between the metatarsalgia and control groups.

Toth and colleagues[12] examined the effect of first ray shortening in the development of second through fifth ray metatarsalgia after metatarsal osteotomy. They found a highly positive correlation between metatarsalgia of the second ray and shortening of the first ray. They found that a greater degree of shortening of the first metatarsal was more likely to cause transfer metatarsalgia in the second through fourth rays, and the severity of pain increased with increased shortening.

In a similar fashion, Jung and colleagues[24] performed a series of dorsiflexion and shortening osteotomies of the first metatarsal in a cadaver model. They first removed a 5-mm base dorsal closing wedge, followed by a 5-mm base plantar closing wedge (creating an overall 5-mm shortening osteotomy). They then removed 1 more 5-mm bone block, to attain a total of 10 mm overall metatarsal shortening. In their results, all 3 procedures resulted in significant decreases in the plantar pressure under the first metatarsal head as compared with the intact foot. Similarly, after all 3 procedures, there was a significant increase in the plantar pressure beneath the second metatarsal head as compared with the intact foot. They also found an increase in plantar pressure under the third and fourth metatarsal head after the 5-mm and 10-mm shortening osteotomies. All of these results were statistically significant.

Taking all of this into account precludes one to think that the simple fact of a patient having a relatively long second metatarsal does not necessarily predispose one to metatarsalgia. It is, however, the relative lengthening of the second metatarsal owing to a short or insufficient first ray that is more the contributing factor to metatarsalgia. When treating patients with metatarsalgia, specifically owing to first ray insufficiency, it is important to determine the underlying cause of metatarsalgia. Shoewear modifications and other nonoperative interventions can be used for symptom management. As with all other pathologic conditions in orthopedics, the root cause must be identified in order to fully resolve the issue. Care must also be taken when treating patients with hallux valgus or hallux rigidus. One must be cautious not to create a relatively long second metatarsal by iatrogenically shortening or malpositioning the first ray.

REFERENCES

1. Maceira E, Monteagudo M. Transfer metatarsalgia post hallux valgus surgery. Foot Ankle Clin N Am 2014;19:285–307.
2. Espinosa N, Maceira E, Myerson M. Current concept review: metatarsalgia. Foot Ankle Int 2008;29(8):871–9.
3. Hardy R, Clapham J. Observations on hallux valgus: based on a controlled series. J Bone Joint Surg Br 1951;33-B:376–91.
4. Steele M, Johnson K, DeWitz M, et al. Radiographic measurements of the normal adult foot. Foot Ankle 1980;1(3):151–8.
5. Coughlin MJ, Jones CP. Hallux valgus: demographics, etiology, and radiographic assessment. Foot Ankle Int 2007;28(7):759.
6. Deschamps K, Birch I, Desloovere K, et al. The impact of hallux valgus on foot kinematics: a cross-sectional, comparative study. Gait Posture 2010;32:102–6.
7. Dietze A, Bahlke U, Martin H, et al. First ray instability in hallux valgus deformity: a radiokinematic and pedobarographic analysis. Foot Ankle Int 2013;34(1):124–30.
8. Maestro M, Besse JL, Magusa M, et al. Forefoot morphotype study and planning method for forefoot osteotomy. Foot Ankle Clin 2003;8:695–710.
9. Slullitel G, Lopez V, Calvi JP, et al. Effect of first ray insufficiency and metatarsal index on metatarsalgia in hallux valgus. Foot Ankle Int 2016;37(3):300–6.
10. Kaipel M, Krapf D, Wyss C. Metatarsal length does not correlate with maximal peak pressure and maximal force. Clin Orthop Relat Res 2011;469:1161–6.
11. Vora AM, Myerson MS. First metatarsal osteotomy nonunion and malunion. Foot Ankle Clin 2005;10:35.
12. Toth K, Huszanyik I, Kellermann P, et al. The effect of first ray shortening in the development of metatarsalgia in the second through fourth rays after metatarsal osteotomy. Foot Ankle Int 2007;28(1):61–3.
13. DiPreta J. Metatarsalgia, lesser toe deformities, and associated disorders of the forefoot. Med Clin North Am 2014;98:233–51.
14. King C, Hamilton G, Ford L. Effects of the lapidus arthrodesis and chevron bunionectomy on plantar forefoot pressures. J Foot Ankle Surg 2014;53:415–9.
15. Cancilleri F, Mariozzi A, Martinelli N, et al. Comparison of plantar pressure, clinical, and radiographic changes of the forefoot after biplanar Austin osteotomy and triplanar Boc osteotomy in patients with mild hallux valgus. Foot Ankle Int 2008;29:817–24.
16. Vandeputte G, Dereymaeker G, Steenwerckx A, et al. The Weil osteotomy of the lesser metatarsals: a clinical and pedobarographic follow-up study. Foot Ankle Int 2000;21(5):370–4.
17. Trask D, Ledoux W, Whittaker E, et al. Second metatarsal osteotomies for metatarsalgia: a robotic cadaveric study on the effect of osteotomy plane and metatarsal shortening on plantar pressure. J Orthop Res 2014;32(3):385–93.
18. Chowdhary A, Drittenbass L, Stern R, et al. Technique tip: simultaneous first metatarsal lengthening and metatarsophalangeal joint fusion for failed hallux valgus surgery with transfer metatarsalgia. Foot Ankle Surg 2017;23(1):e8–11.
19. Maskill J, Bohay D, Anderson J. Gastrocnemius recession to treat isolated foot pain. Foot Ankle Int 2010;31(1):19–23.
20. Herzenberg J, Lamm B, Corwin C, et al. Isolated recession of the gastrocnemius muscle: the Baumann procedure. Foot Ankle Int 2007;28(11):1154–9.

21. Pinney S, Hansen S, Sangeorzan B. The effect on ankle dorsiflexion of gastrocnemius recession. Foot Ankle Int 2002;23:26–9.
22. Chimera N, Castro M, Manal K. Function and strength following gastrocnemius recession for isolated gastrocnemius contracture. Foot Ankle Int 2010;31(5): 377–84.
23. Dreeben S, Noble P, Hammerman S, et al. Metatarsal osteotomy for primary metatarsalgia: radiographic and pedobarographic study. Foot Ankle 1989;9(5): 214–8.
24. Jung HG, Zaret D, Parks B, et al. Effect of first metatarsal shortening and dorsiflexion osteotomies on forefoot plantar pressure in a cadaver model. Foot Ankle Int 2005;26(9):748–53.

Gastrocnemius Recession in the Setting of Metatarsalgia
The Baumann Procedure

Gastón Slullitel, MD*, Juan Pablo Calvi, MD

KEYWORDS

- Metatarsalgia • Gastrocnemius recession • Baumann procedure

KEY POINTS

- Gastrocnemius contracture assessment must be performed when evaluating patients with metatarsalgia.
- Baumann procedure allows for selective lengthening of the gastrocnemius.
- Baumann procedure could be performed in the setting of concomitant procedure without altering patient positioning.

INTRODUCTION

Metatarsalgia is a frequent complaint in patients searching for foot attention. The term refers to localized or generalized forefoot pain in the region of the metatarsal heads.[1] An essential etiologic component of metatarsalgia is the repetitive loading of a locally concentrated force in the forefoot during gait.[2] In the setting of an isolated gastrocnemius contracture, foot biomechanics compensate for decreased ankle dorsiflexion by increased recruitment of extensor digitorum longus and extensor halluces longus during the swing phase of the gait. This muscle recruitment shifts weight-bearing pressure from the hind foot to the forefoot, increasing mechanical stress in this area.[3–5]

If metatarsalgia is considered an entity more than a symptom, evaluation of gastrocnemius contracture must be a part of the physical examination, and, perhaps, gastrocnemius recession alone or in combination with other procedures should be considered as an alternative when treating these patients.

The literature for the use of any gastrocnemius recession technique in the setting of metatarsal pain is, however, far from robust.

The purpose of this article is to review the contribution of gastrocnemius shortening in the occurrence of metatarsalgia and the rationale for the Baumann gastrocnemius recession technique as part of the treatment.

Disclosure Statement: The authors have nothing to disclose regarding this publication.
Department of Foot and Ankle Surgery, J Slullitel Institute of Orthopedics, San Luis 2534, Rosario 2000, Santa Fe, Argentina
* Corresponding author.
E-mail address: gastonslullitel@gmail.com

IMPACT OF GASTROCNEMIUS CONTRACTURE IN THE GENESIS OF METATARSALGIA

The triceps surae is a combination of the 2 strong plantar flexors of the ankle: the gastrocnemius and the soleus muscles. The gastrocnemius originates on the posterior femoral condyles, while the soleus originates on the posterior aspect of the tibia, fibula, and interosseous membrane. Both muscles insert into the calcaneal tuberosity via the Achilles tendon and can contribute to an equinus contracture.[6]

Cavagna and colleagues[7] studied the influence of stretching on muscular strength. The contraction of a previously stretched muscle develops a higher force than if the muscle is previously at rest. The stretching of a muscle requires energy, which is stored as elastic energy in the tissue. When the contraction occurs, the force is amplified and the mechanical efficiency is increased. In the case of a biarticular muscle, stretching varies with the positions of the articulations during contraction at an equivalent energy cost.

During the stance phase of the gait, as with any muscle, the gastrocnemius is tensioned when its attachment is more distant. But as a biarticular muscle, this happens when both the knee is in extension and the ankle in dorsiflexion.

Few studies have examined and defined ankle equinus. Root[8] stated that ankle dorsiflexion greater than 10° in the extended knee position is necessary for a normal gait pattern. This definition is comprehensible if attention is given to the middle stance phase of the gait cycle.

During the middle stance phase, the body weight shifts ventrally while the knee is fully extended and the gastrocnemius is at its maximum strain.[3,9] Those minimum 10° of ankle dorsiflexion is required to make this process possible.[10–12]

Winter and Yack[13] performed an electromyographic analysis of several lower limb muscles during normal walking. Electromyographic activity of the gastrocnemius muscle is low but rising in the beginning of the ankle dorsiflexion up until the point when the ankle is in a neutral position during the stance phase. This phenomenon points out the passive nature of gastrocnemius stretching.

Clinical consequences of gastrocnemius tightness are notable during the weight-bearing phase of gait. A gastrocnemius contracture that does not allow a minimum ankle dorsiflexion eventually moves the center of pressure under the metatarsal heads and this fact explains the link between gastrocnemius tightness and forefoot symptoms.[4]

The prevalence of isolated gastrocnemius contracture varies. DiGiovanni and colleagues[11] reported 75% of patients in a cohort of 34 patients with symptomatic foot and ankle pathology were found to have an isolated gastrocnemius contracture. Hill[14] studied 209 consecutive new patients presenting with primary foot complaints and found that 176 (96.5%) demonstrated restricted ankle dorsiflexion requiring compensation during gait.

Theoretically, lengthening the gastrocnemius should enhance the passive stretching during gait, making the muscle more efficient. Patients that are painful, do have a limited ankle dorsal flexion, which is needed to allow the storage of energy. Lengthening allows recovering of the missing degrees of dorsal flexion and reduces pain. It should return the patient from a pathologic to a more normal situation in which gastrocnemius muscle becomes efficient again.[4]

CLINICAL EXAMINATION

To choose the correct surgical procedure, the components of the triceps surae contributing to an equinus contracture should be differentiated using the Silfverskiöld maneuver.[15]

The soleus only crosses the ankle and subtalar joints; the gastrocnemius also crosses the knee joint. As such, the excursion of the gastrocnemius and soleus muscles can be differentiated on physical examination.[6] When performing Silfverskiöld test, the examiner passively dorsiflexes the ankle with the patient's knee extended and the subtalar joint held in a neutral position.[15] The patient's knee is then flexed while the examiner continues to dorsiflex the ankle (**Fig. 1**). An improvement in dorsiflexion with the knee flexed is considered a positive test and indicative of an isolated gastrocnemius contracture.[16] The most commonly used criterion to indicate an ICG is less than 10° of dorsiflexion with the knee extended, which improves past neutral with knee flexion.[11,16,17] DiGiovanni and colleagues[11] showed, however, that a cutoff at less than 5° of maximal ankle dorsiflexion with the knee fully extended leads to better reproducibility and reliability compared with a cutoff at 10°.

The Silfverskiöld test has been shown to have a sensitivity of 89% and a specificity of 90% compared with goniometric evaluation.[16]

During clinical examination of a patient with metatarsalgia, passive and active ankle dorsiflexion, Silfverskiöld test, and a thorough inspection of the gait are mandatory in order to rule out or diagnose an isolated gastrocnemius contracture as a possible contributor to a patient's symptoms.

DECISION MAKING

An ideal gastrocnemius recession technique allows a controlled lengthening of the gastrocnemius-soleus complex, with the smallest incision possible and the most comfortable positioning of the patient and without the need of changing positioning to perform further procedures.

Although there are many different techniques described for gastrocnemius lengthening, none of them is a risk-free procedure. The most popular proximal procedures present better aesthetic results and allow an early weight load with relatively short periods of immobilization,[18] but they put at risk the saphenous nerve and the greater saphenous vein.[19,20] Elongation at the level of the tendinous muscle joint presents deficient cosmetic results and the possibility of injuring the sural nerve.[21,22] However, the distal procedures achieve a greater correction of the equine with the risk of over-lengthening and loss of strength of plantar flexion.[23]

THE BAUMANN PROCEDURE

Baumann and Koch[24] described this technique in 1989 for the treatment of patients with cerebral palsy.[25] This procedure consists of a gastrocnemius recession through an incision along the proximal medial calf performed in the interval between the

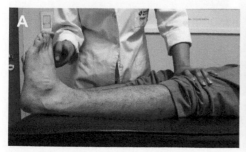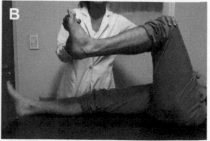

Fig. 1. Silfverskiöld test achieved with the knee extended (*A*) and knee flexed (*B*).

gastrocnemius and soleus fascia.[13] The advantages of the technique are that it isolates the lengthening to the gastrocnemius muscle and preserves muscle strength secondary to the intramuscular lengthening. It is performed in supine decubitus, making it unnecessary to switch the position of the patient when executed in combination with other procedures. Although the original technique is carried on through an 8-cm to 12-cm incision, the authors performed it in a minimally invasive fashion through a 4-cm to 5-cm approach. This theoretically adds cosmesis as another strength.

SURGICAL TECHNIQUE

The patient is placed supine with a bump over the contralateral hip in order to improve medial exposure of the leg. A 4-cm to 5-cm longitudinal incision is made at the midcalf level along the medial aspect of the limb between the junction of the gastrocnemius and soleus muscle bellies. The incision should be placed a 2-cm to 3-cm posterior to the posteromedial edge of the tibia (**Fig. 2**A). Careful dissection is performed in order to identify and retract the greater saphenous vein and saphenous nerve. The crural fascia is then divided longitudinally at the junction of the gastrocnemius and soleus muscles. Careful blunt dissection with the index finger needs to be performed from medial to lateral to separate the plane between the gastrocnemius and soleus muscle bellies (see **Fig. 2**B). Tension is placed on the gastrocnemius muscle by dorsiflexing the ankle joint while keeping the knee fully extended to make the transverse incision across the entire gastrocnemius muscle fascia (see **Fig. 2**C). The intermuscular septum between the medial and lateral heads of the gastrocnemius muscle also is carefully incised (see **Fig. 2**D). If inadequate ankle dorsiflexion is noted (greater than 90°), further recession shall be done separated by 2 cm from each other.

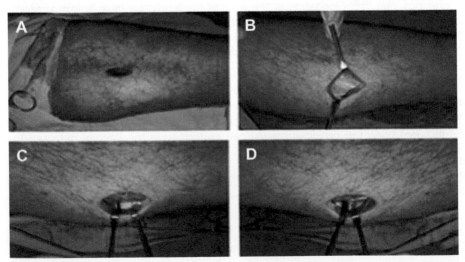

Fig. 2. (*A*) This picture shows the longitudinal incision in the middle level of the calf along the medial aspect of the extremity, 2-cm to 3-cm posterior to the posteromedial edge of the tibia. (*B*) Plane between the gastrocnemius and soleus muscle bellies. (*C*) Transverse incision in the gastrocnemius muscle fascia. (*D*) Gap in the gastrocnemius muscle fascia after the procedure is completed.

POSTOPERATIVE CARE

The procedure itself allows for a short period of immobilization and partial weight bearing according to tolerance in a short walker boot during the first week. A program that includes stretching exercises was initiated according to patient tolerance as soon as the first postoperative week.

In patients in whom an additional procedure was performed, the postoperative immobilization was subdued to the needs of each particular procedure.

During the first postoperative month, a night splint was used to maintain the ankle at 90°.

REHABILITATION PROTOCOL

A supervised physical therapy program was started as soon as possible depending on the underlying pathology, generally during the first postoperative week. The program was composed of eccentric strengthening and myofascial release exercises, work on joint mobility ranges of the ankle and hallux, reeducation of gait, and strengthening and flexibility of the posterior chain.

OUTCOMES

A review of available literature regarding both clinical application and outcome related to gastrocnemius recession revealed little level I or level II evidence and few well-controlled studies. The strength of the evidence greatly varies depending on the indication. Fair evidence-based literature (grade B) exists in favor of gastrocnemius recession as a therapeutic intervention for isolated foot pain due to midfoot to forefoot overload syndrome in adults.[26]

A cadaveric study by Herzenberg and colleagues[25] confirmed the improvement in ankle dorsiflexion associated with a gastrocnemius recession in a cadaveric study using the Baumann procedure. An average of 8° of ankle dorsiflexion was achieved with the knee flexed compared with an average of 14° of ankle dorsiflexion achieved with the knee extended. These results were expected because the 2 recessions of the gastrocnemius muscle had a greater effect on ankle dorsiflexion with the knee extended because this is the anatomic position whereby the gastrocnemius muscle is maximally stretched.

Morales-Muñoz and colleagues[27] studied the effectiveness of proximal gastrocnemius release in treating mechanical metatarsalgia and found a reduction in visual analog scale pain scores and improvement in the American Orthopaedic Foot & Ankle Society scores and average ankle dorsiflexion at 6 months postoperatively in their cohort of 52 patients (78 feet); 36 (69.2%) patients reported satisfaction with the outcome of their surgery, no patients reported worsening of their symptoms after surgery, and 49 of 52 patients returned to active work duty without restriction by 1 month postoperatively.[27]

COMPLICATIONS

Despite the positive operative results, one of the potential drawbacks of a gastrocnemius recession is that mechanical lengthening of the myotendinous unit may contribute to weakness and disability, especially in the athletic population seeking to return to higher demand activities.[18,28,29] Theoretically controlled and selective lengthening of the gastrocnemius-soleus complex or gastrocnemius alone minimizes this weakness, but the literature is still elusive.

In a prospective study that assessed 7 limbs in 4 subjects with isolated gastrocnemius contracture, Chimera and colleagues[28] found significant isometric ($P = .02$) and isokinetic ($P = .01$) strength deficits compared with matched control subjects preoperatively. Three months after the gastrocnemius recession, isometric plantarflexion strength did not change; however, there was a significant increase in isokinetic strength at 60°/s. Although postoperative improvements were noted in the patient group, these values remained below the values of the control subjects, as noted by confidence intervals. Sammarco and colleagues[18] also found that patients remained weaker than their contralateral limb, but that improvements in strength were seen over time.

Although isokinetic testing has been used as the primary outcome measure of muscle performance, it does not effectively capture aspects of muscle performance that may be more demanding and challenging, particularly for sporting activities.[29]

An important concern about the Baumann procedure may be the incision at the medial side of the upper leg.[19,20] This incision could cause potential injury to the saphenous nerve and greater saphenous vein as well as a prominent scar. Careful and blunt dissection of the subcutaneous tissue and the interval between gastrocnemius and soleus is crucial, as well as the use of a retractor in order to fully visualize the fascia over the gastrocnemius to prevent the development of this complication.

Although there are some reports of an endoscopic technique, it is not exempt from nerve damage or loss of plantar flexion strength and requires some surgeon experience. In the series by Phisitkul and colleagues,[22] rates of 3.1% of weakness of plantar flexion and 3.4% of dysesthesia of the sural nerve are reported.

SUMMARY

It is the authors' perspective that the Baumann procedure offers a chance to lengthen the musculotendinous unit in a predictable manner, through a small incision, avoiding the potential risks of over-lengthening the gastrocnemius-soleus complex. A grade B recommendation,[22] appears to be a reasonable convincing evidence to support the use of gastrocnemius recession as a therapeutic intervention for isolated foot pain associated with an over-load syndrome. Consequently, gastrocnemius recession procedures—in this particular case the Baumann technique—might be added to the surgeon's armamentarium when tailoring treatment to each individual patient needs.

REFERENCES

1. Coughlin MJ. Common causes of pain in the forefoot in adults. J Bone Joint Surg Br 2000;82:781–90.
2. Espinosa N, Maceira E, Myerson MS. Current concept review: metatarsalgia. Foot Ankle Int 2008;29(8):871–9.
3. Aronow MS, Diaz-Doran V, Sullivan RJ, et al. The effect of triceps surae contracture force on plantar foot pressure distribution. Foot Ankle Int 2006;27:43–52.
4. Cazeau C, Stiglitz Y. Effects of gastrocnemius tightness on forefoot of during gait. Foot Ankle Clin 2014;19(4):649–57.
5. Cortina RE, Morris BL, Vopat BG. Gastrocnemius recession for metatarsalgia. Foot Ankle Clin 2018;23(1):57–68.
6. Barske HL, DiGiovanni BF, Douglass M, et al. Current concepts review: isolated gastrocnemius contracture and gastrocnemius recession. Foot Ankle Int 2012;33(10):915–21.
7. Cavagna GA, Dusman B, Margaria R. Positive work done by a previously stretched muscle. J Appl Physiol 1968;24(1):21–32.

8. Root L. Varus and valgus foot in cerebral palsy and its management. Foot Ankle 1984;4(4):174–9.
9. Kirby K. Biomechanics of the normal and abnormal foot. J Am Podiatr Med Assoc 2000;90:30–4.
10. Strayer L, Bridgeport M. Recession of the gastrocnemiusdan operation to relieve contracture of the calf muscles. J Bone Joint Surg Br 1950;32:671–6.
11. DiGiovanni C, Kuo R, Tejwani N, et al. Isolated gastrocnemius tightness. J Bone Joint Surg Am 2002;84-A(6):962–70.
12. Jordan R, Cooper M, Schuster R. Ankle dorsiflexion at the heel-off phase of gait: a photokinegraphic study. J Am Podiatr Med Assoc 1964;69:40–6.
13. Winter DA, Yack HJ. EMG profiles during normal human walking: stride-to-stride and inter-subject variability. Electroencephalogr Clin Neurophysiol 1987;67(5): 402–11.
14. Hill R. Ankle equinus: prevalence and linkage to common foot pathology. J Am Podiatr Med Assoc 1995;85(6):295–300.
15. Silfverskiold N. Reduction of the uncrossed two joints muscles of the leg to one joint muscles in spastic conditions. Acta Chir Scand 1924;56:315–30.
16. Patel A, DiGiovanni BF. Association between plantar fasciitis and isolated contracture of the gastrocnemius. Foot Ankle Int 2011;32(1):5–8.
17. DiGiovanni CW, Holt S, Czerniecki JM, et al. Can the presence of equinus contracture be established by physical exam alone? J Rehabil Res Dev 2001; 38:1–7.
18. Sammarco GJ, Bagwe MR, Sammarco VJ, et al. The effects of unilateral gastro-csoleus recession. Foot Ankle Int 2006;27(7):508–11.
19. Kiewiet NJ, Holthusen SM, Bohay DR, et al. Gastrocnemius recession for chronic noninsertional Achilles tendinopathy. Foot Ankle Int 2013;34(4):481–5.
20. Monteagudo M, Maceira E, Garcia-Virto V, et al. Chronic plantar fasciitis: plantar fasciotomy versus gastrocnemius recession. Int Orthop 2013;37(9):1845–50.
21. Thomason P, Baker R, Dodd K, et al. Single event multilevel surgery in children with spastic diplegia: a pilot randomized controlled trial. J Bone Joint Surg Am 2011;93(5):451–60.
22. Phisitkul P, Rungprai C, Femino J, et al. Endoscopic gastrocnemius recession for the treatment of isolated gastrocnemius contracture: a prospective study on 320 consecutive patients. Foot Ankle Int 2014;35(8):747–56.
23. Pinney SJ, Hansen ST Jr, Sangeorzan BJ. The effect on ankle dorsiflexion of gastrocnemius recession. Foot Ankle Int 2002;23(1):26–9.
24. Baumann JU, Koch HG. Ventrale aponeurotische Verlängerung des Musculus gastrocnemius. Operat Orthop Traumatol 1989;1(4):254–8.
25. Herzenberg JE, Lamm BM, Corwin C, et al. Isolated recession of the gastrocnemius muscle: the Baumann procedure. Foot Ankle Int 2007;28:1154–9.
26. Cychosz CC, Phisitkul P, Belatti DA, et al. Gastrocnemius recession for foot and ankle conditions in adults: Evidence-based recommendations. J Foot Ankle Surg 2015;21(2):77–85.
27. Morales-Muñoz P, De Los Santos Real R, Sanz P, et al. Proximal gastrocnemius release in the treatment of mechanical metatarsalgia. Foot Ankle Int 2016;37(7): 782–9.
28. Chimera NJ, Castro M, Manal K. Function and strength following gastrocnemius recession for isolated gastrocnemius contracture. Foot Ankle Int 2010;31:377–84.
29. Nawoczenski DA, Barske H, Tome J, et al. Isolated gastrocnemius recession for achilles tendinopathy: strength and functional outcomes. J Bone Joint Surg Am 2015;97(2):99–105.

Metatarsalgia in Metatarsus Adductus Patients

A Rational Approach

Matthew Varacallo, MD[a],*, Amiethab Aiyer, MD[b]

KEYWORDS

• Metatarsus adductus • Hallux valgus • Foot deformity • Hallux valgus recurrence
• Metatarsalgia

KEY POINTS

- Metatarsus adductus (MA) predisposes patients to hallux valgus (HV), lesser toe deformity, and metatarsalgia.
- Clinical recognition of associated deformities influences operative intervention strategies and algorithmic surgical correction steps to ensure positive patient outcomes.
- While limited long-term follow-up has yet to establish a defined threshold regarding the degree of MA attributed to the increased risk of HV deformity recurrence, an isolated standard distal osteotomy in the setting of severe MA has a high likelihood HV recurrent deformity.

OVERVIEW OF METATARSUS ADDUCTUS

Metatarsus adductus (MA) is a congenital foot condition resulting in adduction of the forefoot at the tarsometatarsal (TMT) joint, medial metatarsal deviation, supination of the hindfoot through the subtalar joint, and a plantarflexed first ray.[1] Whereas consensus regarding the clinical pattern of deformities is well known throughout the literature, it is important to recognize the alternative terminologies that can be used to describe these types of deformities. Other clinical terms used include metatarsus varus, metatarsus adductovarus,[2] metatarsus supinatus, pes adductus, forefoot adductus, and hooked forefoot.[3]

The condition can be seen in association with other intrauterine packaging disorders, with deformity being driven by increased intrauterine pressures during fetal development. MA occurs along a spectrum of deformity and rigidity patterns. Although

Disclosure: The authors report no relevant commercial or financial conflicts of interest or sources of funding.
[a] Department of Orthopaedic Surgery and Sports Medicine, Penn Highlands Healthcare System, 145 Hospital Avenue, Suite 301, DuBois, PA 15801, USA; [b] University of Miami Miller School of Medicine, 900 Northwest 17th Street, Suite 10A, Miami, FL 33131, USA
* Corresponding author.
E-mail address: Matthew.varacallo@gmail.com

the exact underlying pathophysiology remains elusive, there is increasing evidence in the literature highlighting the importance of recognizing MA as an associated deformity pattern that can complicate the management of hallux valgus (HV).[4] We present an overview of the epidemiology, pathomechanics, and comprehensive treatment modalities.

EPIDEMIOLOGY

MA is recognized as the most common congenital foot deformity in newborns.[5] The literature reports an incidence rate of about 1 to 2 cases per 1000 births,[6] although 1 study quoted a rate as high as 3 cases per 1000 births.[7] Although traditional reports in the literature have quoted a lack of gender predilection regarding relative incidence rates,[8] at least 1 recent study has demonstrated an increased rate of MA seen in women.[9] In addition, bilateral involvement occurs in close to half of cases. The overall prevalence is believed to be greater than reported, albeit highly clinician-dependent and sensitive to the particular assessment method used.[10,11]

Intrauterine Development

Several theories have been proposed in reference to contributing risk factors for developing MA. Traditionally, the general consensus in the literature has supported MA as a byproduct of the intrauterine packaging phenomenon.[12] The position of the fetus results in pathologic soft tissue and even osseous development depending on the degree of deformity and force being applied to the developing area of the body.[11] Increasing pressures and compression of the forefoot as the legs are crossed over the body are associated with development of MA. Moreover, as the fetus continues to grow during late gestation, the incidence of MA increases in babies born at full, late, or post term compared with infants delivered before 30 weeks of gestation.[13]

MA can be seen in isolation, although it is not uncommon in association with other conditions that have also been linked to this same intrauterine packaging phenomenon. For example, 1% to 5% of patients with MA also have either developmental dysplasia of the hip or acetabular dysplasia, and up to 10% present with congenital hip dislocation(s).[13] Congenital torticollis can be seen in up to 15% of patients with MA.[5,14] Additional contributing factors to the intrauterine packaging phenomenon include: oligohydramnios, twin pregnancy, and first pregnancy.

PATHOMECHANICS
Metatarsus Adductus and Hallux Valgus

Although the exact cause is not well known, adduction of all of the metatarsals may in part result from muscular imbalances of the tibialis posterior/anterior and the abductor hallucis.[15] The characteristic deformity includes rigidity, a prominent lateral border, difficulty with correction of the foot beyond the midline; these features are more common in pediatric patients.[16] Adults with perseverating MA will often present HV and lesser toe deformities. In addition, patients may present with other deformities of the hindfoot (ie, skew foot, posterior tibial tendon dysfunction, or Charcot-Marie-Tooth disease).[17,18]

There is increasing attention in the literature regarding the potential implications of MA deformity seen in association with HV. The prevalence of MA has been reported to be between 29% and 35% in patients with HV. In general, studies cite up to a 3.5-fold increased risk of development of HV seen in association with MA.[18]

Although the importance of recognizing MA deformity in the setting of HV is becoming more definitively established, the specific nuances and relative impact one condition has on the other (and vice versa) is still somewhat controversial. Currently, the consensus theory is that MA precedes the development of HV deformity.[18] Because all of the metatarsals are adducted in the setting of MA, the notion that MA precedes the development of HV remains plausible.

Medial deviation of the metatarsals leads to attenuation of medial-sided static and dynamic restraints. At the level of the hallux, the abductor hallucis falls plantarward, leaving the medial capsule as the only buttress to metatarsal head deviation. The thin capsule is unable to restrain the metatarsal head and, as it assumes a more varus position, there is a tenodesis effect of the adductor hallucis at its attachment on the proximal phalanx. This leads to valgus deviation of the proximal phalanx, resulting in the extensor hallucis lying lateral to the axis of its mechanical axis. Subsequently, the plantar position of the abductor hallucis, in combination with overpull of the extensor hallucis longus, leads to protonation of the hallux.[18,19]

Development of Metatarsalgia

Considering that all of the metatarsals are medially deviated through the TMT joint apex (**Fig. 1**), there is attenuation of tissues on the medial side of the lesser

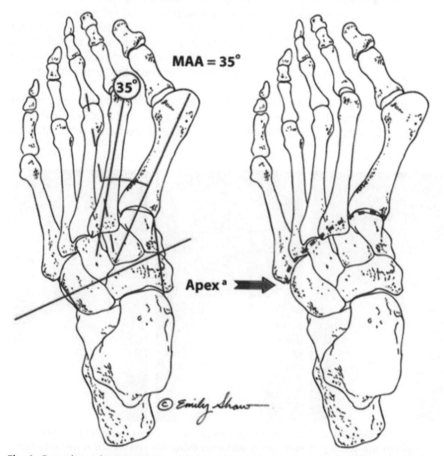

Fig. 1. Dorsolateral tarsometatarsal joint location of the apex of deformity in metatarsus adductus. [a] Apex at the tarsometatarsal (TMT) joints. (© Emily Shaw, MA, CMI, EMT-B 2019 illustrating-medicine.com).

metatarsophalangeal (MP) joints. As the lateral-sided tissues of the MP joints contract, there is a propensity for the lesser toes to migrate laterally, creating a windswept deformity to the toes. This deformity can cause pain and restrict shoe wear. Coronal plane imbalance of the lesser MP joints can lead to sagittal plane imbalance between the flexor and extensor tendons. Overpull of the extensor tendons with a tenodesis effect of the flexor tendons can lead to lesser toe deformities.

Lesser toe deformities are a recognized component of the MA deformity spectrum (**Fig. 2**). The lesser metatarsals normally serve as a buttressing force on the hallux, thus serving as a protective factor against developing HV. MA and lesser toe deformities occur along a deformity spectrum, and severe MA deformity commonly carries with it at least some degree of associated lesser toe deformity. Aiyer and colleagues[19] demonstrated, in a 2016 study, that greater than 50% of patients with severe MA had associated lesser toe deformities. The authors noted the importance for heightened clinical suspicion to appreciate more subtle MA and lesser toe deformities, considering the impact of MA on recurrence of HV deformity after correction.

Dysfunction of the hallucal capability for maintaining appropriate pedal balance of the tripod can lead to transfer metatarsalgia.[20] A retrospective study identified that the 30% of patients with HV undergoing surgery have varying degrees of MA.[9] The presence of HV in the setting of MA can lead to transfer of weight toward to the lesser MP joints. Subsequent attenuation of plantar support structures facilitates sagittal imbalance between the intrinsic/extrinsic musculature.[21]

As a result of these 2 phenomena in the HV patient with MA, patients may present with plantar metatarsal joint pain, callosities over the lesser metatarsal heads, excoriation of the dorsal skin of the proximal interphalangeal joints, corns, and difficulty with

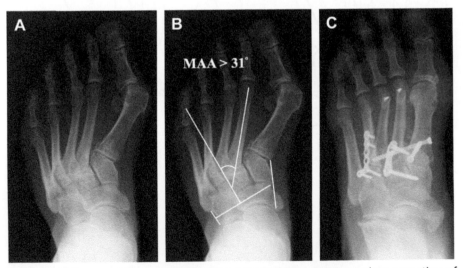

Fig. 2. (*A–C*) Preoperative and postoperative images demonstrate complete correction of hallux valgus in the setting of metatarsus adductus (MA). No recurrence is demonstrated at greater than 1 year of follow-up. This patient with severe MA had a metatarsus adductus angle (MAA) of over 30°. Critical to preventing recurrence in this patient population is correction of the lesser toes. (*Courtesy of Dr Mark Myerson, Miami, FL.*)

fitting into shoes. Shoe wear may also lead to skin breakdown over the medial eminence of the hallux and/or the lesser toes laterally depending on extent of deformity.

RADIOGRAPHIC EVALUATION

Using weight-bearing radiographs of the affected foot, the extent of radiographic severity can be approximated using the MA angle (MAA). There are multiple techniques for evaluating this angle; 1 technique for measuring the MAA is the modified Sgarlato technique. A tangential line along the distal aspect of the medial cuneiform to the most proximal aspect of the navicular is drawn. Similarly, the most proximal and distal aspects of the cuboid (at the lateral aspect of the fifth TMT) are demarcated with a tangential line. A line connecting the midpoint of these 2 lines is drawn. The angle subtended between the bisector of this line relative to the long axis of the second metatarsal is defined as the MAA (**Fig. 3**).

This methodology of delineating the MAA is consistent with the modified Sgarlato method of measuring the MAA.[10] Although several radiographic methods exist to assess MA, the senior author observed high interobserver and intraobserver reliability rates using the modified Sgarlato technique.[9] Although other authors have used the middle cuneiform for ease of radiographic visualization, the senior author has not

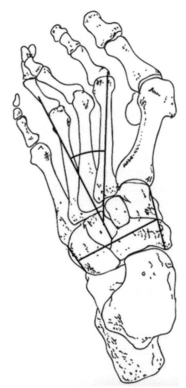

MAA = 27°

Fig. 3. Schematic demonstrating measurement of the metatarsus adductus angle (MAA) using the modified Sgarlato technique. (© Emily Shaw, MA, CMI, EMT-B 2019 illustrating-medicine.com).

had difficulty discerning the lateral aspect of the fifth TMT. The MAA is typically considered abnormal if greater than 20°. Those identified to have MA, were subsequently stratified by the severity of the measured MAA. The deformity was considered mild if the MAA was between 21° and 25°, moderate if the MAA was between 26° and 30°, severe if the MAA was between 31° and 35°, and extremely severe if the MAA was greater than 36°.[9]

The HV angle and intermetatarsal angle (IMA) are also important to evaluate; the latter is of particular importance, because the first to second intermetatarsal space is often collapsed secondary to adduction of the second metatarsal. It is important to account for this when considering surgical intervention.

TREATMENT OPTIONS
Nonoperative Management

The initial management of adult MA deformities is nonoperative treatment modalities, including modifications in shoe wear, metatarsal pads, toe spacers, and protective sleeves for lesser toe deformities. Physical therapy also may be used to facilitate gait training, to help avoid transfer of metatarsalgia-based symptoms.

Operative Management

Algorithm for operative considerations
Recurrence of deformity after HV surgery has been reported to be from 5% to 10%.[22–26] Multiple factors, including inadequate soft tissue releases, technical limitations, and certain patient factors have been implicated. It has been reported that the presence of MA increases the risk for the development of HV. This has been recently corroborated, with recurrence rates as high as 30% in 1 recent study.[19] To best understand the potential effect of MA on HV surgery, it is vital to revisit 3 significant pathoanatomic factors. The first is that persistent adduction of the first metatarsal leads to plantarward displacement of the abductor hallucis. In addition, the thin dorsomedial capsule is unable to appropriately buttress the metatarsal from adducting further. Finally, as the metatarsal head deviates, the adductor halluces tethers the sesamoids/proximal phalanx, and, in combination with the displaced abductor hallucis, the HV deformity is worsened.[27]

Another important point is that adduction of the second metatarsal decreases the first intermetatarsal space. This has 2 effects: first, the specific adduction potentially limits the corrective effect of a distal metatarsal osteotomy because there is limited space for the head to translate laterally. In addition, given that the apex of the MA deformity lies laterally at the TMTs in the coronal plane of an affected foot, there is the potential for under-appreciation for the degree of true deformity that exists at the first intermetatarsal space. This can manifest itself as normal or negative intermetatarsal angle.

Operative management of MA must take into account the adduction of the lesser metatarsals leading to a decreased first and second intermetatarsal space, the degree of true deformity at the first and second intermetatarsal space, and the accompanying lesser toe deformities to prevent recurrence of HV deformity. For HV in the setting of mild to moderate MA, distal, proximal, or modified Lapdius corrections can be undertaken, on the understanding that the rate of radiographic recurrence is 30%.[19] Taking into account the pathoanatomic points mentioned above, an appropriate osteotomy and lesser toe correction can facilitate re-establishment of the buttress mechanism and reduce risk of recurrence (**Figs. 4 and 5**).

The current authors propose the following algorithm to salvage the hallux MP joint, when the MAA is greater than 31° (**Figs. 6 and 7**)

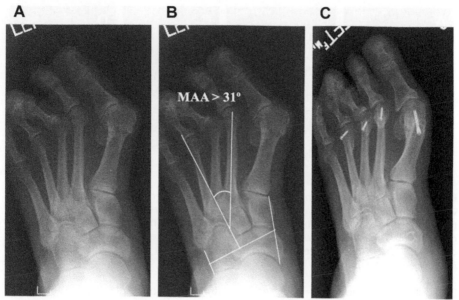

Fig. 4. (*A–C*) Preoperative and postoperative images demonstrate failure of correction of hallux valgus in the setting of metatarsus adductus (MA). In this case, despite attempted correction of the lesser toes, realignment at the apex of deformity has not been completed. As a result, recurrence of hallux valgus is noted in the image on the right. Addressing the entirety of the deformity is critical to preventing recurrence of hallux valgus in the setting of MA. (*Courtesy of Dr Mark Myerson, Miami, FL.*)

1. Unmask the degree of deformity at the first and second intermetatarsal web space. This is accomplished in 1 of 2 ways (a or b):
   a. Second through fourth metatarsal base closing wedge osteotomies
   b. Intra-articular correction with a realignment arthrodesis of the second/third TMTs in the presence of arthritis

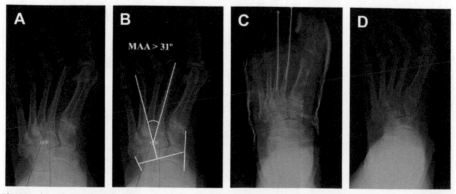

Fig. 5. (*A–D*) Preoperative and postoperative images demonstrate failure of correction of hallux valgus in the setting of metatarsus adductus (MA). In this case, despite attempted correction of the lesser toes, realignment at the apex of deformity has not been completed. As a result, at long-term follow-up (>1 year), recurrence of hallux valgus is noted on the far right. Addressing the entirety of the deformity is critical to preventing recurrence of hallux valgus in the setting of MA. (*Images courtesy of Dr Mark Myerson, Miami, Fl; and /Dr Christopher Narramore.*)

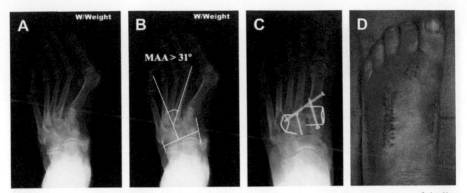

Fig. 6. (*A–D*) Preoperative and postoperative images demonstrate correction of hallux valgus in the setting of metatarsus adductus (MA), without lesser toe correction. A realignment arthrodesis has been completed. No recurrence is demonstrated at greater than 1 year of follow-up. This is a case in which there is risk for recurrence because of lack of correction of the lesser toes, which create an importance buttress effect to the hallux. (*Courtesy of Dr Mark Myerson, Miami, FL.*)

2. Address the wide first and second intermetatarsal angle with a first TMT arthrodesis.
   a. The preoperative first and second intermetatarsal angles may be normal, but metatarsus primus varus gives a hint as to actual deformity in the first webspace
   b. Starting laterally enables one to identify the true degree of deformity at the first and second intermetatarsal space to be visualized (see **Fig. 6**)

Because of the severity of deformity, a more proximal correction is warranted. An arthrodesis of the first TMT is the procedure of choice to reposition the metatarsal head. In conjunction with lateral soft tissue releases around the hallux MP joint, a first TMT arthrodesis will facilitate soft tissue rebalancing around the hallux MP joint. This will aid in prevention of recurrence of HV.

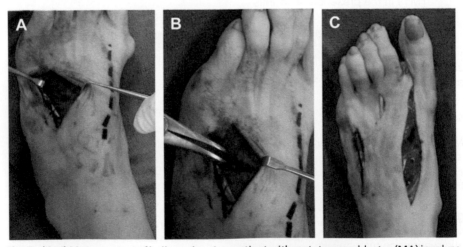

Fig. 7. (*A–C*) Management of hallux valgus in a patient with metatarsus adductus (MA) involves starting dorsolaterally at the apex of deformity. This facilitates unmasking the deformity that exists at the first to second intermetatarsal space. Complete alignment of the foot, including the first ray can be accomplished in this way. (*Courtesy of Dr Mark Myerson, Miami, FL.*)

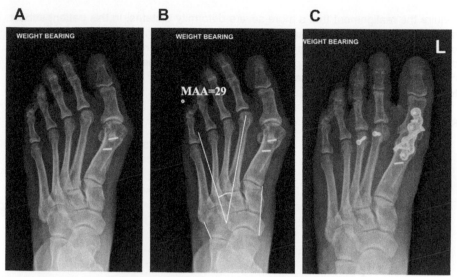

Fig. 8. (*A–C*) Management of the hallux valgus recurrence in the patient with metatarsus adductus (MA) using hallux MP arthrodesis. The MAA was 29°. A distal metatarsal osteotomy was used to treat the HV; note the windswept deformity of the lesser toes. Complete alignment of the foot, including the first ray can be accomplished in this way.

3. Evaluate and treat lesser toe deformities with realignment osteotomies of the metatarsal heads (Weil or lateral translational).
    a. Evaluation of the lesser toes provides an additional sense of the degree of adduction of the metatarsals when windswept lesser toes are observed (lateral deviation of the proximal phalanges at the level of the MP). In the senior author's experience, lesser toe deformities, including windswept toes, compromise the buttress effect that the lesser toes have on the hallux. As a result, the presence of lesser toe deformities may cause recurrence of HV in patients with MA

An alternative option for managing metatarsalgia and facilitate lesser toe correction is to consider a hallux MP arthrodesis. A successful hallux MP fusion can help prevent recurrence of HV deformity, stabilize the first TMT joint, restore balance to the tripod of the foot and alleviate transfer lesions.[26,28] Lesser toe deformities should be corrected as described above, including metatarsal head osteotomies and hammertoe corrections (**Fig. 8**).

SUMMARY

MA places patients at higher risk for HV deformity, subsequent lesser toe deformity, and metatarsalgia. For patients who undergo operative intervention, we believe that a realignment procedure is necessary to adequately treat all aspects of the deformity that are not achieved by standard HV corrective procedures.

When evaluating a patient for HV, clinicians should be mindful to analyze radiographs for the presence of MA. Radiographs should be also scrutinized for evidence of lesser toe deformity. Although a standard distal osteotomy may be used, symptomatic recurrence may develop. Failure to address lesser toe deformities may increase the risk of recurrence by not re-establishing the buttress effect the lesser toes have on the hallux. Limited long-term follow-up precludes us from defining a threshold point of MA deformity that will lead to persistence of HV deformity. Less severe MA may not require the realignment that a more severe deformity dictates. In this patient subset, standard osteotomies may suffice. However, the pathoanatomical points that have been discussed implicate the need for more aggressive realignment procedures in the setting of severe MA. To prevent recurrence of HV, the underlying MA deformity must be adequately addressed; alternatively a hallux MP arthrodesis may be used to prevent recurrence and alleviate transfer metatarsalgia.

REFERENCES

1. Loh B, Chen JY, Yew AK, et al. Prevalence of metatarsus adductus in symptomatic hallux valgus and its influence on functional outcome. Foot Ankle Int 2015; 36(11):1316–21.
2. Lloyd-Roberts GC, Clark RC. Ball and socket ankle joint in metatarsus adductus varus. (S-shaped or serpentine foot). J Bone Joint Surg Br 1973;55(1):193–6.
3. Rushforth GF. The natural history of hooked forefoot. J Bone Joint Surg Br 1978; 60-B(4):530–2.
4. Houghton GR, Dickson RA. Hallux valgus in the younger patient: the structural abnormality. J Bone Joint Surg Br 1979;61-B(2):176–7.
5. Williams CM, James AM, Tran T. Metatarsus adductus: development of a non-surgical treatment pathway. J Paediatr Child Health 2013;49(9):E428–33.
6. Dietz FR. Intoeing—fact, fiction and opinion. Am Fam Physician 1994;50(6): 1249–59, 1262-1244.
7. Dawoodi AI, Perera A. Radiological assessment of metatarsus adductus. Foot Ankle Surg 2012;18(1):1–8.
8. Lichtblau S. Section of the abductor hallucis tendon for correction of metatarsus varus deformity. Clin Orthop Relat Res 1975;(110):227–32.
9. Aiyer AA, Shariff R, Ying L, et al. Prevalence of metatarsus adductus in patients undergoing hallux valgus surgery. Foot Ankle Int 2014;35(12):1292–7.
10. Dawoodi AI, Perera A. Reliability of metatarsus adductus angle and correlation with hallux valgus. Foot Ankle Surg 2012;18(3):180–6.
11. Bourne M, Varacallo M. Anatomy, bony pelvis and lower limb, foot fascia. In: StatPearls. Treasure Island (FL): StatPearls Publishing; 2019.
12. Kite JH. Congenital metatarsus varus. J Bone Joint Surg Am 1967;49(2):388–97.
13. Fishco WD, Ellis MB, Cornwall MW. Influence of a metatarsus adductus foot type on plantar pressures during walking in adults using a pedobarograph. J Foot Ankle Surg 2015;54(3):449–53.
14. Bordoni B, Varacallo M. Anatomy, head and neck, sternocleidomastoid muscle. In: StatPearls. Treasure Island (FL): StatPearls Publishing; 2019.
15. Morcuende JA, Ponseti IV. Congenital metatarsus adductus in early human fetal development: a histologic study. Clin Orthop Relat Res 1996;(333):261–6.
16. Marshall N, Ward E, Williams CM. The identification and appraisal of assessment tools used to evaluate metatarsus adductus: a systematic review of their measurement properties. J Foot Ankle Res 2018;11:25.
17. Berg EE. A reappraisal of metatarsus adductus and skewfoot. J Bone Joint Surg Am 1986;68(8):1185–96.
18. Pontious J, Mahan KT, Carter S. Characteristics of adolescent hallux abducto valgus. A retrospective review. J Am Podiatr Med Assoc 1994;84(5):208–18.
19. Aiyer A, Shub J, Shariff R, et al. Radiographic recurrence of deformity after hallux valgus surgery in patients with metatarsus adductus. Foot Ankle Int 2016;37(2): 165–71.

20. Maceira E, Monteagudo M. Transfer metatarsalgia post hallux valgus surgery. Foot Ankle Clin 2014;19(2):285–307.
21. Ellington JK, Anderson RB, Davis WH, et al. Radiographic analysis of proximal interphalangeal joint arthrodesis with an intramedullary fusion device for lesser toe deformities. Foot Ankle Int 2010;31(5):372–6.
22. Coughlin MJ. Hallux valgus. Instr Course Lect 1997;46:357–91.
23. Fokter SK, Podobnik J, Vengust V. Late results of modified Mitchell procedure for the treatment of hallux valgus. Foot Ankle Int 1999;20(5):296–300.
24. Johnson JE, Clanton TO, Baxter DE, et al. Comparison of Chevron osteotomy and modified McBride bunionectomy for correction of mild to moderate hallux valgus deformity. Foot Ankle 1991;12(2):61–8.
25. Kilmartin TE. Revision of failed foot surgery: a critical analysis. J Foot Ankle Surg 2002;41(5):309–15.
26. Mann RA, Thompson FM. Arthrodesis of the first metatarsophalangeal joint for hallux valgus in rheumatoid arthritis. J Bone Joint Surg Am 1984;66(5):687–92.
27. Coughlin MJ. Hallux valgus. J Bone Joint Surg Am 1996;78(6):932–66.
28. Coughlin MJ, Grebing BR, Jones CP. Arthrodesis of the first metatarsophalangeal joint for idiopathic hallux valgus: intermediate results. Foot Ankle Int 2005;26(10): 783–92.

Freiberg's Infraction
Surgical Options

Hans-Jörg Trnka, MD[a],*, Javier Serrano Lara, MD[b]

KEYWORDS

- Feiberg's infraction • Avascular necrosis • Osteotomies • Metatarsal

KEY POINTS

- Core decompression has been successfully used in the femoral head and the talus, and should promote revascularization of necrotic area. Only 2 cases are reported.
- Joint-Sparing metatarsal osteotomies include intra- and extra-articular closing wedge osteotomies. Both techniques are well reported and reveal good results.
- The Weil osteotomy has become more popular for treatment of Freiberg's infraction. It may be considered as modification of a closing wedge osteotomy with better fixation option.
- Joint destructive procedures are less favorable in comparison with joint-preserving procedures.

INTRODUCTION

The treatment of Freiberg disease, also known as Freiberg's infraction, was first described by Freiberg[1] in 1914. He reported on a series of 6 cases with similar flattened and dorsally collapsed metatarsal heads with subsequent degenerative changes of the metatarsophalangeal joint. Of these patients, 4 were treated conservatively and 2 required metatarsophalangeal joint arthrotomy debridement and removal of loose bodies. Whereas Freiberg proposed trauma to be the cause of the condition, Köhler, in 1923, disagreed with this theory.[2] In 1925, Skillern[3] named it an eggshell fracture, and, in 1922, Panner[4] described it as a peculiar disease of the metatarsal.

The onset of Freiberg's disease is usually between the 11th and 17th year of age, but it also has been noticed in older patients. It is the only osteochondrosis that dominantly affects women, with a reported female-to-male ratio of 5.1. The second

Disclosure: There is no relationship with a commercial company that has a direct financial interest in subject matter or materials discussed in article or with a company making a competing product.
a Foot and Ankle Center, Alserstrasse 43/8d, Vienna 1170, Austria; b Trauma and Orthopaedic Department, Hospital de Rengo, 331, Callejón El Rodeo 97, Rengo, Región del Libertador Gral. Bernardo O'Higgins, Chile
* Corresponding author.
E-mail address: trnka@fusszentrum.at

metatarsal is most frequently involved (68%), followed by the third metatarsal (27%), and the fourth (3%). Usually 1 metatarsal on 1 foot is affected.[5,6]

The pathophysiology is still unknown. Multifactorial causes, including trauma, vascular compromise, or the skeletal maturation process, have been mentioned. Furthermore, systemic disorders, such as diabetes mellitus, systemic lupus erythematosus, and hypercoagulability have been linked to Freiberg's disease.[5]

In 1966, Smillie[7] described the classic staging system based on intraoperative observations of the structural changes of the metatarsal heads.

Stage 1: A narrow fissure fracture in the ischemic epiphysis. Cancellous bone surrounding the fracture appears sclerotic. Compared with adjacent metaphyseal bone, the epiphysis shows deficient blood supply.

Stage 2: Absorption of the cancellous bone occurs in the center of the metatarsal head, leading to collapse of the subchondral bone, while the margins and the plantar aspect of the metatarsal head stay intact. This results in an alteration of the contour of the metatarsal head.

Stage 3: Further central bony resorption occurs, the central portion sinks deeper, creating larger projections on either side. The plantar cartilage stays intact.

Stage 4: The central portion of the articular surface has sunk deep enough to fracture the plantar hinge. Peripheral projections have fractures to form loose bodies. Restoration of normal anatomy is no longer possible.

Stage 5: The final stage shows arthrosis with flattening and deformity of the metatarsal head. Only the plantar aspect of the metatarsal head remains intact. Most of the loose bodies have reduced in size and the shaft of the metatarsal is thickened and dense.

Typical complaints that patients present with are localized pain of the involved metatarsal head. The surrounding tissue presents fusiform swelling. The range of motion is reduced, with primarily dorsal bony impingement, and crepitation may be palpated. Symptoms are exacerbated with barefoot walking or walking with high heels or flexible soles.

Standard radiographic evaluation includes anteroposterior and lateral weight-bearing and oblique lateral images of the forefoot. On the oblique lateral film the dorsoplantar extent of the lesion and loose bodies can be identified. Depending on the progression of the infraction, within the first weeks after onset of the symptoms the joint and osseous structures appear normal with the only exception being that the joint space may be widened. With progression of the disease, the dorsal metatarsal head is increasingly flattened and loose bodies may be seen. The joint space narrows with sclerosis of the metatarsal head.

Especially in the early period of the disease, when plain radiographs are inconclusive, MRI can be helpful in detection. Consistent with osteonecrosis, a hypointense signal on T1-weighted images and mixed hypointense and hyperintense signals on T2-weighted images can be seen.

The first step in the treatment of Freiberg's disease is nonoperative management. The goal of nonoperative management is to eliminate acute pain and to minimize deformation of the metatarsal head. The management includes oral analgesics to relieve acute pain. The use of shoes with a stiffer thicker sole, eventually even with a rocker in the sole, will reduce the range of motion in the metatarsophalangeal joint and consecutively offload the diseased area of the metatarsal head.[5,8]

If the patient is not responding to nonoperative management, surgical intervention is indicated. The various different surgical procedures can be categorized into a group of techniques that alter the abnormal physiology and biomechanics of the metatarsal. These techniques include core decompression and corrective osteotomies, such as closing wedge or shortening osteotomies. The second group of procedures include techniques that restore articular congruency or address the arthritic changes in later stages of the Freiberg's deformity, such as debridement, graftings, or arthroplasties.

Core Decompression

Core decompression has been successfully used in bones such as the femoral head and the talus[9,10] to relieve the elevated intraosseous pressure associated with avascular necrosis.[5] This should promote revascularization of the necrotic area before structural changes occur.[10] The reduction of the intraosseous pressure should also lead to pain reduction. Until now only 2 case reports with promising outcome are available. In 1995, Freiberg and Freiberg[11] presented a unique case of bilateral Freiberg's infraction. The left foot was treated by standard means with metatarsal head arthroplasty, partial proximal phalangectomy, and syndactilization to the third toe. The contralateral side became symptomatic 4 months later and was treated with metatarsal head core decompression. After a 5-year follow-up, the patient was pain free, and able to participate actively in athletics without restriction. In 2006, Dolce and colleagues[12] also reported successful treatment. In both reports the pathologic condition was identified at an early stage without structural changes. A 1.1-mm Kirschner wire was used to create multiple holes. However, following the research of Mont and colleagues,[9] instead of a K-wire, a drill should be used because the use of a Kirschner wire might close the pores of the holes and stop the drainage of the intraosseous pressure.

Joint-Sparing Metatarsal Osteotomies

The principle of the closing wedge osteotomy of the metatarsal head is to rotate the intact plantar articular surface of the metatarsal head into the weight-bearing zone. This closing wedge osteotomy can be performed at the site of the lesion in the metatarsal head or extra-articularly.

Intra-articular Closing Wedge

In 1979, Gauthier and Albaz[13] presented a series of 88 cases in 83 patients treated for Freiberg's infraction. Among these, there were 53 cases of a closing wedge osteotomy across the subchondral necrosis to rotate the lower healthy part of the metatarsal head dorsally to replace the necrotic bone. The osteotomy was transfixed with a simple wire. All 88 cases who underwent surgery were followed-up between 3 and 82 months, with an average of 22 months. Of the 53 cases treated with the new technique, only 1 continued to suffer pain (a bilateral case with a good contralateral result). In 35 cases, passive mobility was measured by an independent examiner rather than the surgeon and averaged 80″ of combined flexion and extension. All results remained stable. There were no complications.

Lee and colleagues[14] reviewed a series of 12 patients with an intra-articular dorsal closing wedge osteotomy fixed with polyglycolide pins with an average follow-up of 45 (22–84) months. All patients were satisfied with the surgery and gained 26° (range 5°–60°) of range of motion of the metatarsophalangeal joint. They measured a mean shortening of 1.7 mm (range 1–2 mm). There was 1 delayed union and no other complication.

Helix-Giordanino and colleagues[15] published a series of 30 consecutive patients reviewed at 15 days, 45 days, and 3 months after surgery. After resection of the necrotic area the osteotomy was fixed with 1 or 2 staples. At the average final follow-up of 6.5 years, 28 patients were very satisfied or satisfied. Metatarsal shortening of 2 mm (1–3 mm) on average was measured. There were no nonunions or transfer metatarsalgia. There was 1 case each of metatarsophalangeal joint subluxation and dislocation, and in 3 cases the painful hardware was removed.

Pereira and colleagues[16] published a long-term follow-up on 20 pediatric patients. Fixation was performed with a stainless steel wire loop. After an average follow-up of 23.4 years (range 15–32 years), 16 patients were rated as excellent and 4 as good. There were no complications in this series.

Extra-articular Closing Wedge Osteotomies

In 1999, Chao and colleagues[17] presented a series of 13 patients treated for Freiberg's disease with an extra-articular dorsal closing wedge osteotomy. The loose bodies were removed but the necrotic area was not excised. The osteotomy was fixed with percutaneous k wires and patients were placed in a short-leg walking cast for 4 weeks. After an average follow-up of 40 months (range 28–54 months), 11 patients were rated as excellent or good, 2 patients (1 fair, 1 poor) had pain, especially after prolonged standing or running. There was 1 case of transfer metatarsalgia.

Lee and colleagues[18] reported using a temporary Kirschner wire fixation for extra-articular dorsal closing wedge osteotomy in 13 cases. They noticed a decreased range of motion in all patients, but all returned to their previous occupational activities. All osteotomies healed within an average of 7 weeks and no complications were encountered. The same technique was used by Capar and colleagues.[19] In their series of 19 patients, 3 were rated poor. Two of those 3 were Smillie classification stage 5. A short-leg cast was applied for 4 weeks.

A series of 10 patients, after an extra-articular dorsal closing wedge osteotomy with an average follow of 36.5 (range 21–66) months, was presented in 1989 by Kinnard and Lirette.[20] They initially fixed the osteotomy using cerclage wires, but because of tendon irritation switched to absorbable sutures. Pain relief was achieved in all patients without any complications. The average shortening was approximately 2.3 mm. Suture fixation of the extra-articular dorsal closing wedge osteotomy was also described by Ikoma and colleagues[21] in a series of 13 feet. They used a nonabsorbable Polyblend suture (FiberWire suture; Arthrex. Inc, Naples, FL, USA). Postoperative management included splint immobilization for 1 week followed by transition to full weight-bearing within 3 weeks. They noted a significant reduction of pain and improvement of the range of motion. No complications were observed.

Weil Osteotomy for Freiberg's Infraction

Using the Weil osteotomy for Freiberg's infraction is a modification of the original Gauthier intra-articular closing wedge osteotomy with excision of the necrotic area. In this modification the wedge apex is more proximal with a more horizontal cut to allow easier screw fixation.

In 2011, Edmondson and colleagues[22] presented a series of 17 patients treated with the Weil osteotomy for symptomatic Freiberg's infraction. Postoperatively, patients were weight-bearing only on the heel for 6 weeks. A significant improvement of the American Orthopaedic Foot & Ankle Society (AOFAS) score was observed: 77% of the patients were rated as excellent and good. In 1 patient, degeneration of the joint increased and a hemiphalangectomy was performed. The same technique was performed by Kim and colleagues[23] in 19 patients. Weight-bearing after surgery was allowed as tolerated in a hard-soled surgical shoe. Postoperative complication included transfer metatarsalgia in 3 cases, and a floating toe and a stiff toe in 1 case each. There was a significant increase of the AOFAS score, the visual analog scale (VAS), and the range of motion of the metatarsophalangeal joint. In 2016, Lee and colleagues[24] performed Weil and dorsal closing wedge osteotomy of the second metatarsal in 15 feet of 15 patients. They reviewed the patients at an average follow-up of 47 months (range 36–72 months). The mean postoperative shortening of the metatarsal length was 3.2 mm. The mean VAS and AOFAS scores were 7.2 and 52.4 points preoperatively, and 2.1 and 78.2 points at 24 months, respectively ($P < .05$). The mean range of motion of the metatarsophalangeal joint increased from 29.4° preoperatively to 46.5° postoperatively ($P < .05$).

Interpositional Arthroplasties

In later stages of Freiberg's infraction (Smillie stage 4–5) it can be difficult to restore joint congruity. Because excisional arthroplasty alone results in residual symptoms and deformities that limit activities, interposition of soft tissue has been advocated.[5] Various donor sites, such as the extensor digitorum longus tendon, the extensor digitorum brevis tendon, a local pedicled extensor hood, the palmaris longus tendon, and the peroneus brevis tendon have been reported.

An interpositional peroneus brevis tendon graft was described by Zgonis and colleagues.[25] They harvested a 3–5-mm-long graft of a third to a half of the peroneus brevis tendon. After debridement of the joint, the free tendon graft is placed on the dorsal aspect of the metatarsophalangeal joint. A Kirschner wire is driven from the toe across the graft into the metatarsal. Patients are permitted partial weight-bearing with crutches and the Kirschner wire is removed after 4 to 6 weeks. No results of this technique have been published. Abdul and colleagues[26] described a rather large series of 25 feet in 23 patients using a local pedicle graft of periosteum and fat as a "Rollmop" spacer for severe Freiberg's infraction. A distal based 4- to 5-cm-long flap of the dorsal capsule of the metatarsophalangeal joint and the dorsal periosteum was rolled around the tip of a nontoothed forceps and sutured into a roll with 2-0 Vicryl. After excisional arthroplasty of the metatarsal head, the graft was positioned into the joint space and sutured down to the plantar plate. VAS and AOFAS scores significantly improved. There was 1 case of superficial wound infection but no transfer metatarsalgia or floating toes.

Grafting

Ajis and colleagues[27] presented an osteochondral distal metatarsal allograft reconstruction as a salvage procedure in 4 cases of late Freiberg's infraction. With an average follow-up interval of 36 months (range 6–66 months), all patients maintained viability of the allograft metatarsal head, and joint radiographs demonstrated osseous union of the metatarsal osteotomy site. No patient had undergone revision surgery. Osteochondral plug transplantation for Smillie stage 3 to 4 was described by Miyamoto and colleagues[28] in 4 cases with an average follow-up of 52 months (range 36–72 months). Using the mosaicplasty autogenous osteochondral grafting system, an osteochondral plug 8.5 mm in diameter and 7.0 mm height was harvested from the lateral aspect of the ipsilateral knee joint. After 4 weeks in a cast, at 6 weeks weight-bearing was allowed. Range of motion of the second metatarsophalangeal joint improved from 19° (range 15° to 25°) before surgery to 40° (range 35° to 45°) at the final follow-up. All patients underwent second-look arthroscopy 1 year after surgery, the International Cartilage Repair Society Assessment Score was normal in 2 patients and nearly normal in another 2 patients. There was no donor site morbidity or local complication.

Joint Debridement

Both open and arthroscopic joint debridement have been reported in the literature. Open joint debridement is a simple procedure with good results. Hoskinson[29] reviewed a group of 12 patients treated surgically for Freiberg's infraction. Four patients had open debridements, 4 metatarsal head excisions, and 4 underwent hemiphalangectomies. The best results were seen in the group who underwent joint debridements. Erdil and colleagues[30] presented 14 patients (8 women and 6 men) with Freiberg's disease Smillie stages IV and V who underwent joint debridement with metatarsal head remodeling. With an average follow-up of 40.2 months (range 14–54 months) the AOFAS and 36-item Short Form Health Survey scores increased significantly.

Only case reports are available for arthroscopic debridement. Carro and colleagues[31] presented a case of arthroscopic joint debridement and excision of the base of the proximal phalanx with a good clinical result. Maresca and colleagues[32] and Hayashi and colleagues[33] described arthroscopic debridement and retrograde drilling of the lesion.

DISCUSSION

Freiberg's infraction is a rare pathologic condition of the lesser metatarsophalangeal joints. In a systematic literature review in 2015, Schade[6] identified 38 publications on surgical treatment of Freiberg's infraction with at least 12 months follow-up. Of these 38 publications, 22 were case series and 16 case reports. Results of a total of 314 patients and 326 feet were reported. Complete resolution in pain and return to full activity was noted in 90% of the performed surgeries. A total of 59 complications were reported, including persistent pain (30), joint stiffness (9), floating toes (5), transfer metatarsalgia (4), weak dorsiflexion (2), hardware irritation (2) and painful scar (2).

The results of joint destructive procedures are less favorable in comparison with joint-preserving procedures. Complete resolution of pain and full return to activities is described in approximately 70% of the joint destructive procedures, whereas after joint-preserving procedures this was achieved in more than 90% of cases.

Over recent decades, the method of fixation for osteotomies has improved. Although in the beginning, percutaneous Kirschner wire fixation and wire loops caused hardware irritations and made hardware removals necessary, more restricted postoperative weight-bearing was also recommended. More recently, the modified Weil osteotomies with screw fixation made more weight-bearing possible in the postoperative period.

Only case reports are available for osteochondral plugs and arthroscopic techniques, thus larger series and prospective or even randomized studies comparing the established techniques should be performed.

REFERENCES

1. Freiberg AH. Infraction of second metatarsal bone. A typical injury. Surg Gynecol Obstet 1914;19:191.
2. Köhler A. Typical disease of the second metatarsophalangeal joint. Am J Radiol 1923;10:705–10.
3. Skillern PG. Eggshell fracture of the metatarsal head. AnnSurg 1915;61(371):372.
4. Panner HJ. A peculiar characteristic metatarsal disease. Acta Radiol 1921;1(1):319–33.
5. Carmont MR, Rees RJ, Blundell CM. Current concepts review: Freiberg's disease. Foot Ankle Int 2009;30(2):167–76.
6. Schade VL. Surgical management of Freiberg's infraction: a systematic review. Foot Ankle Spec 2015;8(6):498–519.
7. Smillie IS. Treatment of Freiberg's infraction. Proc R Soc Med 2019;60(1):29–31.

8. Seybold JD, Zide JR. Treatment of Freiberg disease. Foot Ankle Clin 2018;23(1): 157–69.
9. Mont MA, Schon LC, Hungerford MW, et al. Avascular necrosis of the talus treated by core decompression. J Bone Jt Surg Br 1996;78(5):827–30.
10. Pierce TP, Jauregui JJ, Elmallah RK, et al. A current review of core decompression in the treatment of osteonecrosis of the femoral head. Curr Rev Musculoskelet Med 2015;8(3):228–32.
11. Freiberg AA, Freiberg RA. Core decompression as a novel treatment for early Freiberg's infraction of the second metatarsal head. Orthopedics 1995;18(12):1177–8.
12. Dolce M, Osher L, McEneaney O, et al. The use of surgical decompression as treatment for avascular necrosis of the second and third metatarsal head. Foot 2006;17:162–7.
13. Gauthier G, Elbaz R. Freiberg's infraction: a subchondral bone fatigue fracture. A new surgical treatment. Clin Orthop Relat Res 1929;142:93–5.
14. Lee SK, Chung MS, Baek GH, et al. Treatment of Freiberg disease with intra-articular dorsal wedge osteotomy and absorbable pin fixation. Foot Ankle Int 2007;28(1):43–8.
15. Helix-Giordanino M, Randier E, Frey S, et al. Treatment of Freiberg's disease by Gauthier's dorsal cuneiform osteotomy: retrospective study of 30 cases. Orthop Traumatol Surg Res 2015;101(6 Suppl):S221–5.
16. Pereira BS, Frada T, Freitas D, et al. Long-term follow-up of dorsal wedge osteotomy for pediatric Freiberg disease. Foot Ankle Int 2016;37(1):90–5.
17. Chao KH, Lee CH, Lin LC. Surgery for symptomatic Freiberg's disease: extraarticular dorsal closing-wedge osteotomy in 13 patients followed for 2–4 years. Acta Orthop Scand 1999;70(5):483–6.
18. Lee HJ, Kim JW, Min WK. Operative treatment of Freiberg disease using extra-articular dorsal closing-wedge osteotomy: technical tip and clinical outcomes in 13 patients. Foot Ankle Int 2013;34:111–6.
19. Capar B, Kutluay E, Mujde S. Dorsal closing-wedge osteotomy in the treatment of Freiberg's disease. Acta Orthop Traumatol Turc 2007;41:136–9 [in Turkish].
20. Kinnard P, Lirette R. Dorsiflexion osteotomy in Freiberg's disease. Foot Ankle 1989;9:226–31.
21. Ikoma K, Maki M, Kido M, et al. Extra-articular dorsal closing-wedge osteotomy to treat late-stage Freiberg disease using polyblend sutures: technical tips and clinical results. Int Orthop 2014;38:1401–5.
22. Edmondson MC, Sherry KR, Afolayan J, et al. Case series of 17 modified Weil's osteotomies for Freiberg's and Köhler's II AVN, with AOFAS scoring pre- and post-operatively. Foot Ankle Surg 2011;17(1):19–24.
23. Kim J, Choi WJ, Park YJ, et al. Modified Weil osteotomy for the treatment of Freiberg's disease. Clin Orthop Surg 2012;4:300–6.
24. Lee HS, Kim YC, Choi JH, et al. Weil and dorsal closing wedge osteotomy for Freiberg's disease. J Am Podiatr Med Assoc 2016;106(2):100–8.
25. Zgonis T, Jolly GP, Kanuck DM. Interpositional free tendon graft for lesser metatarsophalangeal joint arthropathy. J Foot Ankle Surg 2005;44:490–2.
26. Abdul W, Hickey B, Perera A. Functional outcomes of local pedicle graft interpositional arthroplasty in adults with severe Freiberg disease. Foot Ankle Int 2018; 39(11):1290–300.
27. Ajis A, Seybold JD, Myerson MS. Osteochondral distal metatarsal allograft reconstruction: a case series and surgical technique. Foot Ankle Int 2013;34:1158–67.
28. Miyamoto W, Takao M, Uchio Y, et al. Late-stage Freiberg disease treated by osteochondral plug transplantation: a case series. Foot Ankle Int 2008;29:950–5.

29. Hoskinson J. Freiberg's disease: a review of the long-term results. Proc R Soc Med 1974;67:106–7.
30. Erdil M, Imren Y, Bilsel K, et al. Joint debridement and metatarsal remodeling in Freibergs infraction. J Am Podiatr Med Assoc 2013;103(3):185–90.
31. Carro LP, Golano P, Farinas O, et al. Arthroscopic Keller technique for Freiberg disease. Arthroscopy 2004;20(Suppl 2):60–3.
32. Maresca G, Adriani E, Falez F, et al. Arthroscopic treatment of bilateral Freiberg's infraction. Arthroscopy 1996;12:103–8.
33. Hayashi K, Ochi M, Uchio Y, et al. A new surgical technique for treating bilateral Freiberg disease. Arthroscopy 2002;18:660–4.

Brachymetatarsia
One-stage Versus Two-Stage Procedures

André Perin Shecaira, MD[a],*,
Rodrigo Mota Pacheco Fernandes, MD[b],[1]

KEYWORDS

• Brachymetatarsia • Metatarsal lengthening • Metatarsalgia • Bone lengthening

KEY POINTS

• Brachymetatarsia is a deformity that usually is cosmetically displeasing and can also become a cause of pain.

• One-stage lengthening of a short metatarsal with or without autogenous or homogeneous bone grafting is a procedure that only requires a single main procedure.

• Two-stage surgery with external fixation (distraction osteogenesis) is preferred for lengthening more than 1.5 cm.

• Single-stage lengthening with a bone graft is associated with fewer complications and faster healing times than callus distraction procedures.

• Combined procedures with gradual lengthening might reduce complications.

ANATOMIC FACTORS

The metatarsal heads are aligned in a parabolic arch in a normal foot, as described by Lelievre.[1–8] This alignment allows the 5 metatarsals to be at the same distance from the ground during weight bearing. In cases of a metatarsal shortening, the transverse metatarsal ligament is stretched, potentially altering the contact of the forefoot with the floor and possibly causing excessive pressure in the forefoot.[9]

For diagnostic purposes, brachymetatarsia is a shortening of the metatarsal superior to 5 mm. This measurement is obtained through weight-bearing radiographs of both feet. The relative length of each metatarsal can be determined by Maestro

Disclosure: The authors have nothing to disclose.
[a] Instituto Nacional de Traumatologia e Ortopedia, Rio de Janeiro, Brazil; [b] CALO - Centro de Alongamento Ósseo, Rio de Janeiro, Brazil
[1] Present address: Avenida das Américas 3301, Bloco 05, Sala 221, Barra da Tijuca, Rio de Janeiro, Rio de Janeiro CEP 22631-003, Brazil.
* Corresponding author. Avenida das Américas 3301, Bloco 05, Sala 221, Barra da Tijuca, Rio de Janeiro, Rio de Janeiro CEP 22631-003, Brazil.
E-mail address: andreshecaira@yahoo.com.br

Foot Ankle Clin N Am 24 (2019) 677–687
https://doi.org/10.1016/j.fcl.2019.08.010
1083-7515/19/© 2019 Elsevier Inc. All rights reserved.

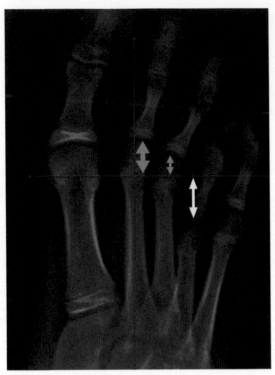

Fig. 1. Maestro criteria for measurement of the metatarsal length; there is a geometric progression of the lesser metatarsals by a factor of 2. Vertical red line is mid-diaphysial to the second metatarsal. Horizontal redline is perpendicular to the vertical red line and passes through the lateral sesamoid. Blue arrows show normal progression and yellow arrow a shortening of the fourth metatarsal.

criteria, with an expected decline in geometric progression of the lesser metatarsals by a factor of 2 (**Fig. 1**).[10]

CLINICAL PRESENTATION

Because this deformity can coexist with other skeletal and systemic abnormalities, a thorough patient physical examination is necessary. For this reason, all these patients should receive a careful multidisciplinary approach, especially when the deformity is present in patient committed with other syndromes.

Even though pain is a possible symptom, the most usual patient concern involves the cosmetic appearance the foot. In most cases, the feet are pain free and the major worry is about the appearance of the foot.[9]

However, there may be a dorsally displaced corresponding toe, which can produce callosities and make the fitting of shoes difficult. Transfer metatarsalgia is also a possible symptom, and, in long-standing deformities, further digital deviation can occur and even lead to formation of a bunion deformity (**Fig. 2**).[11]

In all instances, the Kelikian push-up test should be performed to assess whether the metatarsal-phalangeal joint is flexible and reducible (**Fig. 3**). Its importance is that nonreducible joints need a complete capsular release, sometimes associated with extensor tendon lengthening, before any bone surgery, which implies more invasive surgery and worse foot function after treatment.[12]

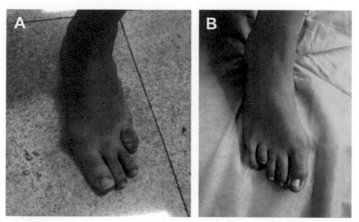

Fig. 2. (*A*) Dorsally displaced fourth digit. (*B*) Long-standing lateral deviation of the toes led to a bunion formation.

NONOPERATIVE TREATMENT

In patients with pain or callosities, the first option of treatment should embrace conservative measures such as medical insoles, orthotics, and wider toe-box shoes. Only when nonoperative measures fail to relive pain or the main complaint is aesthetic should surgery be indicated.[13]

SURGICAL TREATMENT

Multiple acute and gradual lengthening surgical techniques have been described for correction of this type of foot deformity. All techniques try to ensure a better appearance, facilitate shoeing, or solve possible transfer metatarsalgia[11,12](**Fig. 4**).

One-Stage Procedures

One-stage procedures are those that realize an acute lengthening of the metatarsal. In 1969, McGlamry and Cooper[14] first described the lengthening of a short metatarsal in

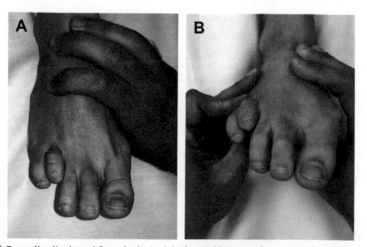

Fig. 3. (*A*) Dorsally displaced fourth digit. (*B*) The Kelikian push-up test showing a nonreducible joint.

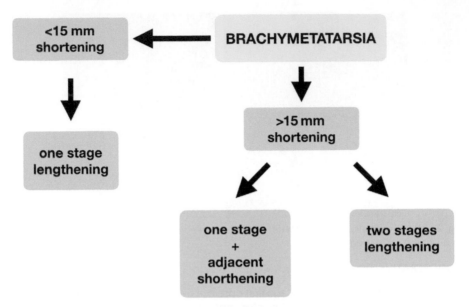

Fig. 4. Algorithm of surgical treatment of brachymetatarsia.

a single surgery using bone graft from the calcaneus to fill the gap obtained after the osteotomy site was acutely spread apart.

Since then, several acute lengthening techniques have been described in procedures using various sites of autogenous bone grafts, allografts, synthetic materials, sliding osteotomies, and many different internal fixation materials.[13]

The main disadvantage of these type of procedures is the limitation of the capacity to lengthen the bone. Acute lengthening has a greater risk when more than 15 mm of gain is attempted, because a large neurovascular stretch done at once might compromise the viability of the toe because of vasospasm. In addition, the soft tissue is placed at great tension, predisposing the patient to metatarsophalangeal dislocations or later joint rigidity.[13,15–17]

When the amount of lengthening is not feasible by interposition bone graft surgery, the usual alternative is to consider associated shortening of adjacent bones. In many instances, by realizing the shortening of adjacent metatarsals and phalanges, the surgeon is able to achieve the targeted parabola, without the need of an external fixator for long periods, making the whole process more comfortable and faster for the patient and reducing associated risks of 2-stage surgery. This benefit is especially useful when brachymetatarsia affects the first metatarsal, because surgeons can easily diminish the lateral rays, needing a smaller 1-stage procedure.[17]

There is no exact amount of shortening recommended in these cases. The amount should be enough that the lengthening needed is less than the limit of a 1 stage procedure –(1.5 cm). Extreme shortening must also be done carefully so that vascular compromise is not an issue.[9,13,17]

Sliding osteotomies
In 1984, Marcinko and colleagues[18] described a Z-shaped sliding osteotomy to treat posttraumatic shortening. The main advantage of this technique is the reduced necessity to use some form of bone graft, thus reducing donor site morbidity and tissue

scaring, which is of great value because the main purpose of the surgery is cosmetic improvement.[19]

When some sort of graft is needed, adjacent metatarsal bone is usually the most favorable donor site. However, sliding osteotomies have very few complications and good functional and cosmetic results[20] (**Fig. 5**).

The literature lacks large studies showing 1-stage lengthening with sliding osteotomies. Most work involves case reports with no complications and good functionality; none show large gains.[18,21–23]

Singh and Dudkiewicz[24] described a prospective cohort series of sliding osteotomies to treat metatarsalgia resulting from iatrogenic first metatarsal shortening. They operated on 16 patients with transfer metatarsalgia after shortening from a Wilson osteotomy to treat hallux valgus. Good pain relief was shown when more than 8 mm of lengthening was obtained.

Bone grafting

Various donor sites for grafts (tibia, iliac bone crest, calcaneus, autologous metatarsal, and so forth) have been reported in this modality of treatment (**Fig. 6**).[15,25,26] All have shown the same limitations: diminished capacity to lengthen the metatarsal and donor site morbidity, for which a promising alternative is the use of homologous bone.[13]

In a systematic review realized by Jones and colleagues,[27] analyzing 349 feet that underwent acute lengthening with bone graft, the mean size gain was 13.3 mm. There was a faster healing index (centimeters per month) and fewer complications than in callus distraction surgery.

Giannini and colleagues[13] used homologous metatarsal bone to graft and acutely lengthened 41 feet. Radiographically, the mean gain was 13 mm, with a 23% increase in size. Overall, no complications were present and full bone union was achieved in every patient.

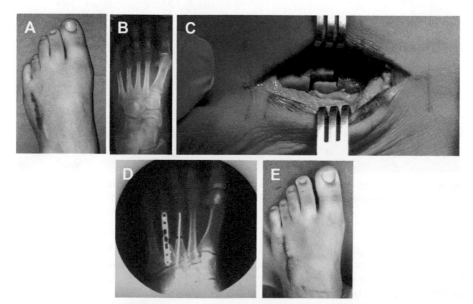

Fig. 5. (*A*) Fourth metatarsal brachymetatarsia with shortening after a failed attempt at gradual lengthening. (*B*) Preoperative radiography. (*C*) Step sliding osteotomy. (*D*) Plate/screw fixation of the lengthening and shortening of the third metatarsal. (*E*) Postoperative clinical result.

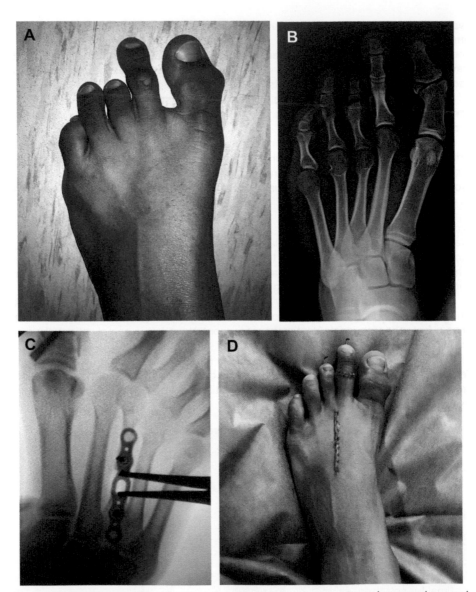

Fig. 6. (A) Shortening of the third metatarsal, with consequent pain under second ray and claw toe. (B) Preoperative radiograph. (C) Lengthening trough bone spreader and (D) clinical result.

In every acute lengthening, concern about soft tissues is needed to avoid joints dislocations, neuromuscular damage, and to optimize stretching capacity. Usually a Z-plasty to elongate extensor tendons, freeing the interosseous muscles, or a flexor tendon tenotomy is undertaken.[9,13,15]

Complications

Besides a possible undercorrection, neurovascular compromise caused by acute lengthening is the main concern in 1-stage procedures; rapid stretching of the blood vessels might lead to vasospasm.[26] However, recent data show that, with the proper freeing of soft tissue and respecting the limit of 15 mm of total gain, this is a rare occurrence.[13,17]

Single-stage lengthening with bone grafting has shown a 19.48% overall rate of complications. Some loss of the range of motion of the metatarsophalangeal joint is the most common and limiting concern. Most studies also report, with less frequency, possible loss of fixation, bone graft resorption, bone deviation, joint subluxation, and graft donor site morbidity.[27]

Two-Stage Procedure

Two-stage procedures involve some sort of osteotomy associated with concomitant bone distraction. Through callotasis, new bone is formed and the short metatarsal gains the desired length after the surgical procedure is complete.[9,28] This technique usually is used when there is a need to overcome the limitations of 1-stage surgery, in which no more than 15 mm of lengthening is desired.[17]

After the osteotomy, the distraction callotasis is usually done with an external fixator at a rate of less than 1 mm/d, allowing bone growth and soft tissues to gradually accommodate, thus reducing the risk of vasospasm caused by acute stretch of the neurovascular bundle.[29,30]

Surgical technique

Most bone distraction surgery is done with a unilateral external fixator to achieve careful placement of 2 pins in the proximal segment and another 2 in the distal segment.[12] To prevent plantar flexion of the lengthened metatarsal, the pins should be placed in a manner so that distraction is done parallel to the ground and not necessarily respecting the anatomic axis of the bone. This point is especially important in the first metatarsal, where a plantar flexion might cause an undesired varus compensatory deformity of the hind foot.[31]

Osteotomy is realized through a small dorsal incision with careful extensor tendon protection. Afterward, after a latency period of about a week (no more than 10 days to avoid premature consolidation), gradual distraction is started[9] (Fig. 7). The same surgery can be executed percutaneously with a bone burr, theoretically preserving more soft tissue and causing better cosmetics.[32]

Pitfalls

In contrast with long bone lengthening, distraction should be done at a slower rate in a metatarsal. When a distraction rate of 0.75 mm/d is undertaken, even though good bone formation is expected, this might be too fast for tendon stretching and can lead to joint rigidity or dislocations.[33] A distraction rate of 0.25 mm twice a day is optimal for soft tissue elongation and bone formation.[34]

To prevent joint dislocation, besides joint stretching and tendon lengthening, surgeons can also fixate the metatarsal-phalangeal joint with a Kirschner wire that is left in the patient until the bone distraction phase is complete.[35] Another option is extending the fixation beyond the metatarsal-phalangeal joint and not invading it, by placing Schanz pins into the proximal phalanx throughout the process.[11]

Complications

Two-stage procedures have a high risk of complications, with more than 50% of the surgeries being involved with some sort of problem. Major complications such as metatarsal malalignment, poor bone formation and joint dislocations occur in about 12.62% of the cases (Fig. 8). Postoperative joint rigidity has a 17% rate of occurrence

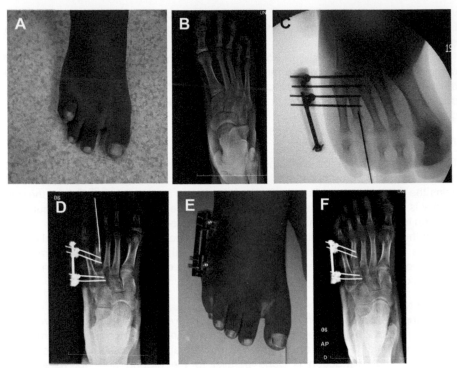

Fig. 7. (A) Fourth metatarsal shortening and (B) preoperative radiograph. (C) External fixator placement and osteotomy. (D) Lengthening of the fourth metatarsal. (E) Postoperative clinical and (F) radiological final result.

and 8% rate of pin tract infection.[27] In 1 series, in which the mean amount of gain was 30%, all patients showed some loss in range of motion (120° before and 57° after surgery on average).[36]

Most studies show that, by respecting a limit of lengthening of no more than 40% of the metatarsal original size, most complications are avoided.[9,31,36] This finding is especially seen when subluxation is in question, with the joint being excessively stressed because of overlengthening.[15,33]

Future Directions

As the techniques of distraction osteogenesis for bone lengthening have evolved, attempts have been made to improve the patients' experiences by reducing the time of external fixation usage. A promising alternative is plating the area after the desired length is achieved, decreasing the fixator time for the patient and guaranteeing a faster postoperative rehabilitation.[37] However, reports on this topic are limited, and only small series have been undertaken in diverse anatomic locations and in patients of different ages.[38]

Another promising technique was described by Woo and colleagues,[39] who realized an anatomic reconstruction of fourth brachymetatarsia with 1-stage iliac bone and cartilage cap grafting. Instead of a mid-diaphysis osteotomy, the dissection and spreading was taken into the metatarsal-phalangeal joint space, reconstructing the joint and gaining length. In theory, this has the advantage that, by dissection through the joint space, it is possible to achieve a more effective release.

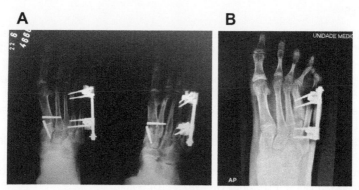

Fig. 8. (*A*) Poor bone formation in a gradual lengthening of the fourth metatarsal. (*B*) Bone malalignment and metatarsal-phalangeal joint dislocation in a fourth metatarsal gradual lengthening.

With a capsulotomy and the plantar plate incision, there is no need for a wider subperiosteal dissection, avoiding a decrease in the circulation and thus permitting wider bone spreading.

In 56 operated feet, they showed a 22.9-mm gain on average, with only 1 case of nonunion and no neurovascular complications. Thirteen patients complained of loss of range of motion but did not require secondary surgery.

Authors' Experience

The authors have a case series of 12 operated feet, with lengthening of 13 metatarsals, in which only 1 patient had a 1-stage procedure done because of having less than 1.5 cm of shortening. The remaining patients underwent gradual lengthening with monolateral external fixator.

Mostly there was a very low incidence of complication; mainly superficial pin tract infection solved with topical or oral antibiotics. In 1 case of lengthening of 2 adjacent metatarsals, the foot developed acute compartment syndrome during bone stretching and decompression was necessary. There was also a case of delayed bone formation, and since then we have tried not to exceed a bone distraction rate of 0.75 mm/d.

Whenever possible (no active pin tract infection), the authors use plating to shorten the fixator usage period.

SUMMARY

Brachymetatarsia is a rare deformity with controversial clinical presentation. Because most patients seek medical attention because of the cosmetic appearance of the foot, it is hard to decide when and how to intervene. Smaller and less aggressive procedures (most 1-stage surgeries) have a limited capacity to gain the total desired length and involves the risk of donor site morbidity. However, gradual distraction makes lengthening of more than 1.5 cm possible, but requires the use of an external fixator and the procedures cause many complications. In all instances, adjacent metatarsal shortening should be combined to diminish exposure to excessive lengthening, selecting 1-stage or 2-stage surgeries based on each patient's deformities, concerns, and clinical needs.

REFERENCES

1. Lee KB, Park HW, Chung JY, et al. Comparison of the outcomes of distraction osteogenesis for first and fourth brachymetatarsia. J Bone Joint Surg Am 2010;92: 2709–18.
2. Bartolomei FJ. Surgical correction of brachymetatarsia. J Am Podiatr Med Assoc 1990;80(2):76–82.
3. Handelman RB, Perlman MD, Coleman WB. Brachymetatarsia: a review of the literature and case report. J Am Podiatr Med Assoc 1986;76:413–6.
4. Tachdjian MO. Pediatric orthopedics. 2nd edition. Philadelphia: WB Saunders; 1990. p. 2633–7.
5. Takakura Y, Tanaka Y, Fujii T, et al. Lengthening of short great toes by callus distraction. J Bone Joint Surg Br 1997;79(6):955–8.
6. Urano Y, Kobayashi A. Bone-lengthening for shortness of the fourth toe. J Bone Joint Surg Am 1978;60(1):91–3.
7. Wakisaka T, Yasui N, Kojimoto H, et al. A case of short metatarsal bones lengthened by callus distraction. Acta Orthop Scand 1988;59(2):194–6.
8. Lelie'vre J. Pathologie du pied [Pathology of the foot]. Paris: Masson; 1971.
9. Schimizzi A, Brage M. Brachymetatarsia. Foot Ankle Clin 2004;9:555–70.
10. Besse JL. Metatarsalgia. Orthop Traumatol Surg Res 2017;103(1S):S29–39.
11. Lamm BM. Percutaneous distraction osteogenesis for treatment of brachymetatarsia. J Foot Ankle Surg 2010;49(2):197–204.
12. Lamm BM. Metatarsal lengthening. In: Rozbruch RS, Ilizarov S, editors. Limb lengthening and reconstruction surgery. 1st edition. New York: Informa Healthcare; 2007. p. 291–302.
13. Giannini S, Faldini C, Pagkrati S, et al. One- stage metatarsal lengthening by allograft interposition: a novel approach for congenital brachymetatarsia. Clin Orthop Relat Res 2010;468:1933–42.
14. McGlamry ED, Cooper CT. Brachymetatarsia: a surgical treatment. J Am Podiatry Assoc 1969;59(7):259–64.
15. Baek GH, Chung MS. The treatment of congenital brachymetatarsia by one-stage lengthening. J Bone Joint Surg Br 1998;80:1040–4.
16. Desai A, Lidder S, Armitage AR, et al. Brachymetatarsia of the fourth metatarsal, lengthening scarf osteotomy with bone graft. Orthop Rev 2013;5:e21.
17. Kim HT, Lee SH, Yoo CI, et al. The management of brachymetatarsia. J Bone Joint Surg Br 2003;85-B:683–90.
18. Marcinko DE, Rappaport MJ, Gordon S. Posttraumatic brachymetatarsia. J Foot Surg 1984;23:45 1–453.
19. Kosaka M, Sugimoto H, Kamiishi H. A rare case of unilateral brachymetatarsia of the 2nd toe. Cong.Anom 1993;33:357–61.
20. Chairman EL, Dallalio AE, Mandracchia VJ. Brachymetatarsia IV ; A different surgical approach. J Foot Surg 1985;24:361–3.
21. Tabak B, Lefkowitz H, Steiner I. Metatarsal-slide lengthening without bone grafting. J Foot Surg 1986;25:50–3.
22. Sinclair GG, Shoemaker SK, Seibert SR. Iatrogenic brachymetatarsia. J Foot Surg 1991;30:580–4.
23. Solomon MG, Blacklidge DK. Brachymetatarsia: case report and surgical considerations. J Am Podiatr Med Assoc 1995;85:685–9.
24. Singh D, Dudkiewicz I. Lengthening of the shortened first metatarsal after Wilson's osteotomy for hallux valgus. J Bone Joint Surg Br 2009;91(12):1583–6.

25. Kashuk KB, Hanft JR, Schabler JA, et al. Alternative autogenous bone graft donor sites in brachymetatarsia reconstruction: a review of the literature with clinical presentations. J Foot Surg 1991;30:246–52.

26. Alter SA, Feinman B, Rosen RG. Chevron bone graft procedure for the correction of brachymetatarsia. J Foot Ankle Surg 1995;34:200–5.

27. Jones MD, Pinegar DM, Rincker SA. Callus distraction versus single-stage lengthening with bone graft for treatment of brachymetatarsia: a systematic review. J Foot Ankle Surg 2015;54:927–31.

28. Ilizarov GA, Deviatov AA, Trokhova VG. Surgical lengthening of the shortened lower extremities. Vestn Khir Im I I Grek 1972;108(2):100–3.

29. Levine SE, Davidson RS, Dormans JP, et al. Distraction osteogenesis for congenitally short lesser metatarsals. Foot Ankle Int 1995;16(4):196–200.

30. Davidson RS. Metatarsal lengthening. Foot Ankle Clin 2001;6(3):499–518.

31. Shim JS, Park SJ. Treatment of brachymetatarsia by distraction osteogenesis. J Pediatr Orthop 2006;26:250–4.

32. Barreiro GC, Garcia AG, Dominguez JMG. Percutaneous foot surgery for the treatment of brachymetatarsia: a case report. Foot Ankle Surg 2017;23(3):e1–5.

33. Kawashima T, Yamada A, Ueda K, et al. Treatment of brachymetatarsia by callus distraction (callotasis). Ann Plast Surg 1994;32:191–9.

34. Choi IH, Chung MS, Baek GH, et al. Metatarsal lengthening in congenital brachymetatarsia: one-stage lengthening versus lengthening by callotasis. J Pediatr Orthop 1999;19:660–4.

35. Peña-Martínez VM, Palacios-Barajas D, Blanco-Rivera JC, et al. Results of external fixation and metatarsophalangeal joint fixation with K-wire in brachymetatarsia. Foot Ankle Int 2018;39(8):942–8.

36. Masada K, Fujita S, Fuji T. Complications following metatarsal lengthening by callus distraction for brachymetatarsia. J Pediatr Orthop 1999;19:394–7.

37. Iobst CA, Dahl MT. Limb lengthening with submuscular plate stabilization: a case series and description of the technique. J Pediatr Orthop 2007;27:504–9.

38. Oh CW, Baek SG, Kim JW, et al. Tibial lengthening with a submuscular plate in adolescents. J Orthop Sci 2015;20(1):101–9.

39. Woo SH, Bang CY, Ahn HC, et al. Anatomical reconstruction of the fourth brachymetatarsia with one-stage iliac bone and cartilage cap grafting. J Plast Reconstr Aesthet Surg 2017;70(5):666–72.

Resection Arthroplasty
Current Indications and Tips

Javier Z. Guzman, MD[a,b], Ettore Vulcano, MD[a,b,*]

KEYWORDS

• Resection arthroplasty • Rheumatoid arthritis • Plantar foot pain • Metatarsalgia

KEY POINTS

• Resection arthroplasty is a salvage procedure for refractory cases of metatarsalgia.
• Patients older than 50 years of age with rheumatoid arthritis may be better candidates than those younger than 50 years of age and without rheumatoid arthritis.
• Recurrence of hallux valgus deformity, in the setting of resection arthroplasty, may be minimized by performing fusion of the first metatarsophalangeal joint.

INTRODUCTION

Metatarsalgia is a common cause of plantar forefoot pain, generally affecting the area of the distal metatarsal (MT) in one, some, or all of the rays from the second through the fourth ray. The cause may be multifactorial, but it can be categorized into primary (intrinsic anatomic variations of the MTs and MTs relationship to the foot), secondary (inflammatory arthropathies, hallux rigidus, malalignment secondary to trauma), or iatrogenic.[1] The complexity of this common problem must be treated on a patient-specific basis, requiring conservative versus surgical treatment. In this review, the authors focus on resection arthroplasty, a relatively less commonly used method for treatment, but nonetheless sometimes required for refractory cases of persistent metatarsalgia.

INDICATIONS

Resection arthroplasty is largely limited to patients with rheumatoid arthritis and to insensate diabetics. In general, patients indicated for this procedure are elderly individuals with poor protoplasm and severe deformities of the lesser toes.[2]

There are several reasons for its restricted use, including transfer lesions to neighboring MTs and significant forefoot instability. Most commonly, the rheumatoid foot

Disclosure Statement: The authors have nothing to disclose.
[a] Mount Sinai West, NYC, 425 West 59th Street 5th Floor, New York, NY 10019, USA; [b] Leni & Peter W. May Department of Orthopedic Surgery, Icahn School of Medicine at Mount Sinai, New York, NY, USA
* Corresponding author. Mount Sinai West, NYC, 425 West 59th Street 5th Floor, New York, NY 10019, USA.
E-mail address: ettorevulcano@hotmail.com

presents with hallux valgus and lesser toe deformities. The pathophysiology includes loss of dorsal bony buttress at the metatarsophalangeal (MTP) joint, with concurrent deterioration of the adjacent soft tissue envelope. Loss of bony buttress causes dorsal subluxation of the interossei leading to dorsal subluxation of the proximal phalanx.[3] In turn, there is weakening and loss of plantar plate integrity over time, causing rupture, which leads to uncovering of the MT heads and disruption of the transverse tie bar and windlass mechanisms.[4] This uncovering of the MT heads along with altered biomechanics leads to significant pain of the plantar forefoot, which may need to be addressed surgically if MT padding and bracing are insufficient. The Larsen grading system for rheumatoid arthritis joint destruction may be used to quantify those patients (Larsen III–V), which may not be amenable to joint-preserving osteotomy correction.[5]

Patients with diabetes have a distinct, but related issue, which is elevated plantar pressure secondary to Charcot architectural changes. Moreover, these patients have prominent MT pads, which are subjected to repetitive trauma and subsequent ulcerations. In cases of refractory ulcerations despite total contact casting, metatarsal resection leads to significant decreases in plantar pressures, and healing response.[6]

SURGICAL TECHNIQUES

Resection arthroplasty for metatarsalgia was first described by Hoffman[7] in 1911 for severe claw and curved toes. He performed resection of the MT heads through a singular plantar incision behind the web of the toes. He described no need to tenotomy of contracted tendons because bone resection was sufficient.

In the 1960s, Clayton[8] described resection arthroplasty through 1 transverse dorsal incision, in which he resected several MT heads with 1 surgical exposure. In this same setting, he described resection of the proximal phalanx base in order to correct cocked up toe deformities. He advised that it is essential to remove the entire MT head and neck to allow the proper seating of the phalanx and MT stump without significant crowding.

Similar to Clayton, Fowler[9] went on to describe a similar technique of resection arthroplasty for rheumatoid patients with severe foot deformities, in which the investigator made a dorsal incision proximal to the web of the toes, with reflection of the skin, vein, and extensor tendons in 1 layer. The proximal phalangeal bases were excised, and MT heads were removed only so much as to straighten the convex anterior line of the metatarsals. The investigator described the lengths of the MTs as being important, noting that the second, third, and fourth MTs are likely to be more prominent, especially when this effect was amplified in patients with a short first MT. In addition, the investigator corrected the distal displacement of the MT pad by making an elliptical skin incision on the plantar surface directly behind the MTs, producing a neo-metatarsal pad in the correct position. Kates and colleagues,[10] using the same concepts as Fowler, developed a technique in which only the MT heads were excised through a generous curved plantar incision. Adherent sesamoids were excised as well, before first MT head resection. The technique called for Kirschner (K)-wire fixation in the hallux to maintain axial alignment. They then performed a 2.5-cm elliptical skin incision similar to Fowler's technique. Although similar to Fowler's description, the advantage is the singular incision as opposed to dual incisions: Kates' technique incorporates the elliptical incision with index exposure incision, which is not possible using Fowler's dorsal incision.

In 1974, Watson[11] reviewed resection arthroplasty performed using the Kates-Kessel-Kay description versus Fowler's technique in patients with and without rheumatoid arthritis and found no distinct advantage in either technique with regards to patient outcomes. However, he made several observations that furthered the understanding of surgical technique and indications. He noted that patients over the age of 50 years with rheumatoid arthritis had favorable outcomes compared with patients who were younger and did not have rheumatoid arthritis. In addition, he noted that MT ends with distal extension greater than their neighbors by more than 1 cm appeared to correspond to increased plantar MT head calluses and presumably pain. In either case, results were less than promising because only 18% of all feet that underwent surgical treatment were pain free.

Mann and Schakel[12] described a modification of previous resection arthroplasty techniques, which included arthrodesis of the first MTP joint. The lesser toes are exposed by making 2 dorsal incisions: one between the second and third MT and the other in the intermetatarsal space between the fourth and fifth toes. They performed circumferential dissection around the MTP joints to release the plantar plate and aponeurosis. These soft tissue releases, allows opening of the joint substantially, and subsequently, resection of the MT head was performed. Resection was aimed plantar and proximal, with enough bone resected to allow the proximal phalanx to lie without tension. Pins were then used to hold the phalanx and MT in place. Before finalizing arthrodesis of the great toe, it was ensured that it did not extend more than 5 mm with respect to the second. If this was the case, then more bone was resected. The investigators demonstrated significant improvements in 90% of patients. The fusion of the great toe increased the overall length of the hallux, which in turn led to earlier liftoff and decreased forces across the lesser toes. Keller resection arthroplasty, which was frequently combined with other resection arthroplasty techniques, led to a shorter hallux, prolonged liftoff, and thus a higher potential of recurrence of callosities and hallux valgus.[13]

More recently, Lui[14] modified Mann's description of resection arthroplasty in an effort to restore sagittal balance of the lesser toes. Incisions are similar in both cases, with subsequent resection of the MT heads; however, at this point a K-wire is inserted into the proximal phalanx base and brought out through the tips of the toes. While being held in the correct transverse plane, the wires are inserted into the MTs until they approach the subchondral bone. The wire is then bent dorsally at the level of the resection to restore sagittal balance at the MTP joint. The hallux is fused in this technique.

AUTHOR'S PREFERRED TECHNIQUE

The senior author attempts preservation of the joints unless severely arthritic or deformed. A Lapidus procedure associated with resection of the lesser MT heads may help correct or prevent hallux valgus deformity without sacrificing the hallux MTP. In case of an arthritic hallux MTP, a fusion is preferred. Inclusion of an interphalangeal joint (IP) may also be considered in patients with clinical signs of arthritis and/ or severe hallux valgus interphalangeus. The IP should otherwise be spared because fusion of both IP and MTP joints may increase overall nonunion rate (20%–30%) as well as having mediocre patient satisfaction postoperatively. Therefore, unless the patient complains of pain at the IP joint, it may be best to avoid or delay the arthrodesis. Although plate and screws are the preferred fixation for the fusion, this is not always possible because of the poor bone quality in rheumatoid patients. In said circumstances, a Steinman pin or threaded K wires may be valuable tools to have available in the operating room. Unless a Lapidus procedure is selected, a longitudinal incision is performed over the hallux MTP to perform the fusion, followed by a transverse incision across the forefoot to expose the lesser MT heads. With such an approach, all extensor tendons are released. The MT heads are then resected at the head-neck junction, beveled at 45° so as to decrease the plantar stress at the remaining MT shaft. Resection of the lesser metatarsals should be included if the toes are irreducible. With respect to healthy adjacent MTP joints, once resection arthroplasty has been performed, it should be carried out to all toes. A shortening osteotomy to the neighboring metatarsals will likely not allow sufficient resection, and the convex anterior line of the MT will not be restored. The disparity in the longer MT may lead to increased stress, which can eventually lead to stress fractures and pain. Once adequate resection has been obtained, all lesser toes are percutaneously pinned to the respective MT to maintain the alignment for 6 weeks. Pin site infection and pin migration with K-wire are relatively low.[15] Strap dressing and K-wire fixation less than 6 weeks have been associated with a deformity recurrence rate of up to 50%.[16,17]

SUMMARY

Resection arthroplasty for painful or ulcerated forefoot deformities is a technique that can provide significant pain relief.[18] However, it should be performed sparingly and limited to patients older than 50 years with rheumatoid arthritis or insensate diabetic feet. Complications are common, and recent studies demonstrate that a significant proportion of patients remain dissatisfied with the results.[19] Complications include recurrence of hallux valgus, recurrence of hammer toes, plantar callosities, and continued pain. Preservation of the MTP joints should always be considered, particularly at the hallux. Hallux valgus deformities in the absence of arthritic changes may be addressed with a Lapidus and either shortening or resection of the lesser metatarsals. Conversely, a hallux MTP, with or without IP fusion, should be considered for all other cases presenting with symptomatic erosive changes.

REFERENCES

1. Espinosa N, Brodsky JW, Maceira E. Metatarsalgia. J Am Acad Orthop Surg 2010;18(8):474–85.
2. Horita M, Nishida K, Hashizume K, et al. Outcomes of resection and joint-preserving arthroplasty for forefoot deformities for rheumatoid arthritis. Foot Ankle Int 2018;39(3):292–9.
3. Molloy AP, Myerson MS. Surgery of the lesser toes in rheumatoid arthritis: metatarsal head resection. Foot Ankle Clin 2007;12(3):417–33, vi.
4. Stainsby GD. Pathological anatomy and dynamic effect of the displaced plantar plate and the importance of the integrity of the plantar plate-deep transverse metatarsal ligament tie-bar. Ann R Coll Surg 1997;79(1):58–68.
5. Larsen A, Dale K, Eek M. Radiographic evaluation of rheumatoid arthritis and related conditions by standard reference films. Acta Radiol Diagn (Stockh) 1977;18(4):481–91.
6. Patel VG, Wieman TJ. Effect of metatarsal head resection for diabetic foot ulcers on the dynamic plantar pressure distribution. Am J Surg 1994;167(3):297–301.
7. Hoffmann P. An operation for severe grades of contracted or clawed toes. 1911. Clin Orthop Relat Res 1997;(340):4–6.
8. Clayton ML. Surgery of the forefoot in rheumatoid arthritis. 1960. Clin Orthop Relat Res 1998;(349):6–8.
9. Fowler AW. A method of forefoot reconstruction. J Bone Jt Surg Br 1959;41-B: 507–13.
10. Kates A, Kessel L, Kay A. Arthroplasty of the forefoot. J Bone Jt Surg Br 1967; 49(3):552–7.

11. Watson MS. A long-term follow-up of forefoot arthroplasty. J Bone Jt Surg Br 1974;56B(3):527–33.
12. Mann RA, Schakel ME 2nd. Surgical correction of rheumatoid forefoot deformities. Foot Ankle Int 1995;16(1):1–6.
13. McGarvey SR, Johnson KA. Keller arthroplasty in combination with resection arthroplasty of the lesser metatarsophalangeal joints in rheumatoid arthritis. Foot Ankle 1988;9(2):75–80.
14. Lui TH. Technical tips: modified resection arthroplasty for correction of rheumatoid forefoot deformity. Foot Ankle Surg 2010;16(2):74–7.
15. Kramer WC, Parman M, Marks RM. Hammertoe correction with k-wire fixation. Foot Ankle Int 2015;36(5):494–502.
16. Klammer G, Baumann G, Moor BK, et al. Early complications and recurrence rates after Kirschner wire transfixion in lesser toe surgery: a prospective randomized study. Foot Ankle Int 2012;33(2):105–12.
17. Holinka J, Schuh R, Hofstaetter JG, et al. Temporary Kirschner wire transfixation versus strapping dressing after second MTP joint realignment surgery: a comparative study with ten-year follow-up. Foot Ankle Int 2013;34(7):984–9.
18. Thomas S, Kinninmonth AW, Kumar CS. Long-term results of the modified Hoffman procedure in the rheumatoid forefoot. Surgical technique. J Bone Joint Surg Am 2006;88(Suppl 1 Pt 1):149–57.
19. Matsumoto T, Kadono Y, Nishino J, et al. Midterm results of resection arthroplasty for forefoot deformities in patients with rheumatoid arthritis and the risk factors associated with patient dissatisfaction. J Foot Ankle Surg 2014;53(1):41–6.

UNITED STATES POSTAL SERVICE®
Statement of Ownership, Management, and Circulation
(All Periodicals Publications Except Requester Publications)

1. Publication Title	2. Publication Number	3. Filing Date
FOOT AND ANKLE CLINICS OF NORTH AMERICA	016 – 368	9/18/2019

4. Issue Frequency	5. Number of Issues Published Annually	6. Annual Subscription Price
MAR, JUN, SEP, DEC	4	$337.00

7. Complete Mailing Address of Known Office of Publication *(Not printer) (Street, city, county, state, and ZIP+4®)*

ELSEVIER INC.
230 Park Avenue, Suite 800
New York, NY 10169

Contact Person: STEPHEN R. BUSHING
Telephone *(Include area code)*: 215-239-3688

8. Complete Mailing Address of Headquarters or General Business Office of Publisher *(Not printer)*

ELSEVIER INC.
230 Park Avenue, Suite 800
New York, NY 10169

9. Full Names and Complete Mailing Addresses of Publisher, Editor, and Managing Editor *(Do not leave blank)*

Publisher *(Name and complete mailing address)*

TAYLOR BALL, ELSEVIER INC.
1600 JOHN F KENNEDY BLVD. SUITE 1800
PHILADELPHIA, PA 19103-2899

Editor *(Name and complete mailing address)*

LAUREN BOYLE, ELSEVIER INC.
1600 JOHN F KENNEDY BLVD. SUITE 1800
PHILADELPHIA, PA 19103-2899

Managing Editor *(Name and complete mailing address)*

PATRICK MANLEY, ELSEVIER INC.
1600 JOHN F KENNEDY BLVD. SUITE 1800
PHILADELPHIA, PA 19103-2899

10. Owner *(Do not leave blank. If the publication is owned by a corporation, give the name and address of the corporation immediately followed by the names and addresses of all stockholders owning or holding 1 percent or more of the total amount of stock. If not owned by a corporation, give the names and addresses of the individual owners. If owned by a partnership or other unincorporated firm, give its name and address as well as those of each individual owner. If the publication is published by a nonprofit organization, give its name and address.)*

Full Name	Complete Mailing Address
WHOLLY OWNED SUBSIDIARY OF REED/ELSEVIER, US HOLDINGS	1600 JOHN F KENNEDY BLVD. SUITE 1800 PHILADELPHIA, PA 19103-2899

11. Known Bondholders, Mortgagees, and Other Security Holders Owning or Holding 1 Percent or More of Total Amount of Bonds, Mortgages, or Other Securities. If none, check box ▶ ☐ None

Full Name	Complete Mailing Address
N/A	

12. Tax Status *(For completion by nonprofit organizations authorized to mail at nonprofit rates) (Check one)*
The purpose, function, and nonprofit status of this organization and the exempt status for federal income tax purposes:
☒ Has Not Changed During Preceding 12 Months
☐ Has Changed During Preceding 12 Months *(Publisher must submit explanation of change with this statement)*

PS Form **3526**, July 2014 *(Page 1 of 4 (see instructions page 4))* PSN: 7530-01-000-9931 PRIVACY NOTICE: See our privacy policy on www.usps.com

13. Publication Title	14. Issue Date for Circulation Data Below
FOOT AND ANKLE CLINICS OF NORTH AMERICA	JUNE 2019

15. Extent and Nature of Circulation			Average No. Copies Each Issue During Preceding 12 Months	No. Copies of Single Issue Published Nearest to Filing Date
a. Total Number of Copies *(Net press run)*			256	270
b. Paid Circulation *(By Mail and Outside the Mail)*	(1)	Mailed Outside-County Paid Subscriptions Stated on PS Form 3541 *(Include paid distribution above nominal rate, advertiser's proof copies, and exchange copies)*	144	164
	(2)	Mailed In-County Paid Subscriptions Stated on PS Form 3541 *(Include paid distribution above nominal rate, advertiser's proof copies, and exchange copies)*	0	0
	(3)	Paid Distribution Outside the Mails Including Sales Through Dealers and Carriers, Street Vendors, Counter Sales, and Other Paid Distribution Outside USPS®	68	86
	(4)	Paid Distribution by Other Classes of Mail Through the USPS *(e.g., First-Class Mail®)*	0	0
c. Total Paid Distribution *(Sum of 15b (1), (2), (3), and (4))*			212	250
d. Free or Nominal Rate Distribution *(By Mail and Outside the Mail)*	(1)	Free or Nominal Rate Outside-County Copies Included on PS Form 3541	33	5
	(2)	Free or Nominal Rate In-County Copies Included on PS Form 3541	0	0
	(3)	Free or Nominal Rate Copies Mailed at Other Classes Through the USPS *(e.g., First-Class Mail)*	0	0
	(4)	Free or Nominal Rate Distribution Outside the Mail *(Carriers or other means)*	0	0
e. Total Free or Nominal Rate Distribution *(Sum of 15d (1), (2), (3) and (4))*			33	5
f. Total Distribution *(Sum of 15c and 15e)*			245	255
g. Copies not Distributed *(See Instructions to Publishers #4 (page #3))*			11	15
h. Total *(Sum of 15f and g)*			256	270
i. Percent Paid *(15c divided by 15f times 100)*			86.53%	98.04%

* If you are claiming electronic copies, go to line 16 on page 3. If you are not claiming electronic copies, skip to line 17 on page 3.

16. Electronic Copy Circulation	Average No. Copies Each Issue During Preceding 12 Months	No. Copies of Single Issue Published Nearest to Filing Date
a. Paid Electronic Copies ▶		
b. Total Paid Print Copies (Line 15c) + Paid Electronic Copies (Line 16a) ▶		
c. Total Print Distribution (Line 15f) + Paid Electronic Copies (Line 16a) ▶		
d. Percent Paid (Both Print & Electronic Copies) (16b divided by 16c × 100) ▶		

☒ I certify that 50% of all my distributed copies (electronic and print) are paid above a nominal price.

17. Publication of Statement of Ownership

☒ If the publication is a general publication, publication of this statement is required. Will be printed in the DECEMBER 2019 issue of this publication. ☐ Publication not required.

18. Signature and Title of Editor, Publisher, Business Manager, or Owner

Stephen R. Bushing Date 9/18/2019

STEPHEN R. BUSHING - INVENTORY DISTRIBUTION CONTROL MANAGER

I certify that all information furnished on this form is true and complete. I understand that anyone who furnishes false or misleading information on this form or who omits material or information requested on the form may be subject to criminal sanctions (including fines and imprisonment) and/or civil sanctions (including civil penalties).

PS Form **3526**, July 2014 *(Page 3 of 4)* PRIVACY NOTICE: See our privacy policy on www.usps.com

Moving?

Make sure your subscription moves with you!

To notify us of your new address, find your **Clinics Account Number** (located on your mailing label above your name), and contact customer service at:

Email: journalscustomerservice-usa@elsevier.com

800-654-2452 (subscribers in the U.S. & Canada)
314-447-8871 (subscribers outside of the U.S. & Canada)

Fax number: 314-447-8029

Elsevier Health Sciences Division
Subscription Customer Service
3251 Riverport Lane
Maryland Heights, MO 63043

*To ensure uninterrupted delivery of your subscription, please notify us at least 4 weeks in advance of move.

ELSEVIER

Printed and bound by CPI Group (UK) Ltd, Croydon, CR0 4YY

03/10/2024

01040482-0010